Visibly Different

Coping with disfigurement

Edited by

Richard Lansdown PhD FBPsS CPsychol
Honorary Senior Lecturer
Institute of Child Health, University of London, UK

Nichola Rumsey BA(Hons) MSc PhD CPsychol AFBPsS
Principal Lecturer in Psychology, University of the West of England, UK

Eileen Bradbury BSocSc PGCE DipCOT PhD
Health Psychologist in Plastic Surgery, Lecturer in Health Psychology
University of Manchester, UK

Tony Carr BSc PhD DClinPsychol CPsychol AFBPsS
Head of Clinical Teaching Unit
Psychology Department, University of Plymouth, UK

James Partridge MA(Oxon) MSc
Director of Changing Faces, London, UK
Visiting Research Fellow, University of the West of England, UK

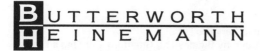
BUTTERWORTH
HEINEMANN

Butterworth-Heinemann
Linacre House, Jordan Hill, Oxford OX2 8DP
A division of Reed Education and Professional Publishing Ltd

ℛ A member of the Reed Elsevier plc group

OXFORD BOSTON JOHANNESBURG
MELBOURNE NEW DELHI SINGAPORE

First published 1997

British Library Cataloguing in Publication Data

A catalogue record for this book is available from the British Library

Library of Congress Cataloguing in Publication Data

A catalogue record for this book is available from the Library of Congress

ISBN 0 7506 3424 3

Typeset by Keyword Typesetting Services Ltd
Printed and bound in Great Britain by Biddles Ltd, Guildford and King's Lynn

Contents

Contributors

Nick Ambler BSc MSc CPsychol
Nick Ambler works as a clinical psychologist in the Regional Burns and Plastic Surgery Service in Frenchay Hospital, Bristol. His main interests are the psychological effects of trauma and altered appearance, pain and chronic illness.

Eileen Bradbury BSocSc PGCE DipCOT PhD
Eileen Bradbury is a health psychologist in the Department of Plastic and Reconstructive Surgery, at the Withington Hospital, Manchester. She has recently completed a PhD on the psychological aspects of disfigurement of the face, head and hands.

Tony Carr BSc PhD DClinPsychol CPsychol AFBPsS
Tony Carr is Head of the Clinical Teaching Unit in the Psychology Department at the University of Plymouth. His special interests are assessment in clinical practice and the matching of treatment to particular needs.

David Harris LRCP MRCS MB BS FRCS MS
David Harris is the Senior Consultant Plastic Surgeon and founder of the Sub-regional Plastic Surgery and Burns Unit, Derriford Hospital, Plymouth. His particular interests include paediatric plastic surgery and cosmetic surgery. His research into the symptomatology of abnormal appearance has done much to establish the importance of cosmetic surgery as an effective intervention to relieve psychological distress and dysfunction.

Daniela Hearst BSc (Hons) MPhil AFBPs S CPsychol
Daniela Hearst is a consultant clinical psychologist at Great Ormond Street Hospital for Children, working in the Craniofacial Unit. Her particular interests include psychological factors influencing the timing of surgical interventions and long-term follow-up of children with single suture cranio-synostosis. She is currently working for a PhD on self-concept and attachment in children with mild and severe craniofacial anomalies.

Richard Lansdown PhD FBPsS CPsychol
Richard Lansdown was a consultant psychologist at Great Ormond Street Hospital for Children for over 20 years. He is now attached to the Centre for International Child Health at the University of London Institute of Child Health and is the Adviser for Education at the Partnership for Child Development, University of Oxford. His most recent book is *Children in Hospital* (Oxford University Press, 1996).

Judith Middleton MSc PhD CPsychol
Judith Middleton is a consultant clinical psychologist in the Department of Clinical Neuropsychology at The Radcliffe Infirmary, Oxford. Her particular area of interest is working with children with craniofacial disfigurement and in child clinical neuropsychology.

Tim Moss BSc(Hons)
Tim Moss is a postgraduate researcher in the Department of Psychology, University of Plymouth. He is currently involved in a project with Tony Carr and David Harris on the clinical need and psychological process in response to disfigurement and is working towards a PhD as part of this project.

Poppy Nash BA(Hons) LCST PhD
Poppy Nash originally trained as a speech and language therapist, and now works in the Work Skills Centre, Department of Psychology, University of York. She has recently completed a PhD in the area of cleft lip and palate. Her book, *Living with Disfigurement: psychosocial implications of being born with a cleft lip and palate* (Avebury) was published in 1995.

James Partridge MA(Oxon) MSc
James Partridge is the Founder Director of the UK Charity, Changing Faces (launched in 1992), which provides help for children and adults who have facial disfigurements and seeks to raise public awareness about this issue. He is the author of the book *Changing Faces: the Challenge of Facial Disfigurement* (Penguin, 1990) and has written and spoken widely on the subject. He suffered severe burns at the age of 18 years, and, after university, he worked as a health economist and teacher as well as running a dairy farm.

Dai Roberts-Harry BDS MSc FDS DOrth MOrth
Dai Roberts-Harry is a consultant orthodontist at the Leeds Dental Institute. His interest lies in the area of patients with cleft lip and palate.

Emma Robinson BSc MSc
Emma Robinson is a postgraduate researcher, based at the University of the West of England, working with James Partridge and Nichola Rumsey evaluating outcomes of interventions provided by the charity Changing Faces.

Nichola Rumsey BA(Hons) MSc PhD CPsychol AFBPsS
Nichola Rumsey is a principal lecturer in psychology, at the University of the West of England. Her PhD examined the psychological problems

associated with facial disfigurement. She was coauthor (with Ray Bull) of the book, *The Social Psychology of Facial Appearance* (Springer-Verlag, 1988).

Elizabeth Walters MB ChB MRCPsych
Elizabeth Walters is a consultant child and adolescent psychiatrist at The Park Hospital for Children, Oxford, and the Oxford Craniofacial Unit, Radcliffe Infirmary, Oxford.

Additional contributors:

Sarah Bishop
Sarah Bishop was formerly a researcher in the Cleft Lip and Palate Research Team, Department of Psychology, University of Sheffield. She now teaches in Catalunya.

William Shaw BDS MScD PhD FDSRCS DOrth RCS DDorth
William Shaw is Professor of Orthodontics at the Turner Dental School, University Dental Hospital, Manchester.

Introduction

Richard Lansdown and Nichola Rumsey

There are over 400 000 people in the UK with a scar, blemish or deformity that severely affects their ability to lead a normal life (Office of Population Censuses and Surveys, 1988).

The genesis of this book occurred in Cambridge in 1989 when two psychologists (Richard Lansdown and Nichola Rumsey) met a plastic surgeon (David Harris) at a meeting of the British Association of Aesthetic Plastic Surgeons. They ruefully discussed the lack of attention, funding and research concerning the care of those with visible disfigurements. They made vague plans to meet again and to convene a multidisciplinary group of like-minded people who might work together, sharing ideas and experiences. Unlike many such plans, this one took off and the Disfigurement Interest Group was founded.

The numbers grew and the group attracted professionals from a variety of disciplines, including speech and language therapy, clinical psychology, health psychology, plastic surgery, orthodontics and psychiatry, and from the newly founded charity, Changing Faces.

After three or four years of biannual meetings to exchange ideas and discuss research, fifteen 'core' members took the decision to write a book. This decision seemed logical for a variety of reasons. Such a project would provide a framework for the group's activities and would be a way of harnessing the group's knowledge and experience. It was also a response to the clear need to publish an authoritative account of the problems and issues in the field of visible disfigurement.

The process of writing was a mixture of democratic discussions and mild autocracy. Everyone concerned put forward views on the structure and content. We eventually concluded that we wanted to write three separate, small volumes: one to consist of accounts of what it is like to be disfigured; another to summarize the relevant research literature; and a third to discuss service provision and ways of offering help to those with a visible disfigurement. We compromised with the present three-section format, in the hope that some readers would be able to use these as a complete volume and to allow readers to focus on the stand-alone sections. We continue to speculate on the value of separate publications.

In order to complete the task, two managing editors (Richard Lansdown and Nichola Rumsey) and three Section Editors (James Partridge, Tony Carr and Eileen Bradbury) were appointed and chapters allocated according to interest. Early drafts were circulated to everyone so that all main contributors could have a sense of ownership of the book as a whole. The mild autocracy came from the section editors in forming the separate chapters into coherent wholes, and from the managing editors who carried out a final edit to ensure a more or less consistent style and level of clarity. Although time consuming, this method has ensured as much coherence and agreement as possible, a task that has, in most instances, been surprisingly easy.

In the final chapter we have pulled together the themes that have emerged from the book and have suggested ways in which service provision and support for those with a visible difference should develop. We have argued the case for care to be delivered by a co-ordinated multidisciplinary team and we hope that in producing this book we have demonstrated that we, at least, have practised what we preach.

Reference

Office of Population Censuses and Surveys (1988). *Report 1: The prevalence of disability among adults*. London: HMSO.

Section One

The Experience of Being Visibly Different

Edited by James Partridge

Chapter 1

Introduction to Section One

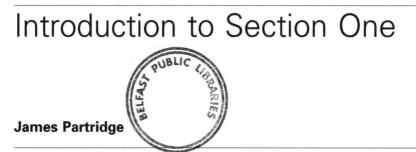

James Partridge

One of my children's favourite books when they were younger was called *Flat Stanley* (Brown, 1968). Stanley Lambchop was a normal child until one day a notice-board fell on him and he became only half an inch thin/thick! He was so flat that he could go under doors and through gratings in the road. 'When Stanley got used to being flat, he enjoyed it... [and he found] that being flat could be helpful.' Of course, it took some getting used to, and wasn't always fun, but Flat Stanley became well known and respected for his unique qualities.

Reading stories of Stanley's escapades to the children was hugely rewarding for me personally because I was able to share with them the experience of being visibly different. My own face and body were badly burned in a fire some twenty-five years ago and, since then, I have had to come to terms with my changed appearance and with other people's reactions to it.

Of course, my children have had to do this too. Like it or not, they have had to learn how to cope with being seen with me in school settings, on the beach, in a restaurant, wherever there are other people around. All fathers are embarrassing but I suspect my children may find me doubly – or even triply! – so. I suspect this is partly because the way that I have developed to manage actively my public reception is deliberately, but (I think) subtly, extrovert. I call it 'proactive' and I have described it in some depth in my book (Partridge, 1990).

The opening section of this present book is intended to give a flavour of what the experience of having a visible difference is like for a larger group of people with a whole variety of disfigurements. In some ways I am surprised that it needs to be written at all, because every human being knows about being 'different' from every other human being. We are all unique after all....

The cultural and personal definitions of visible difference

Our concern here is to explore the human experience of being significantly visibly different compared with a norm, a norm that is either defined for us by the culture or by ourselves. These two meanings of visibly different are crucial to understand from the outset.

First, there is the case of an individual who has some facial or body feature that obtrudes itself onto the gaze of anyone they meet so that they are perceived as 'different' according to some implicit cultural norm (Goffman, 1963). The difference carries with it a stigma that marks out the person involved as socially out of step. Occasionally, the deviation from the norm renders to the person a high social regard, as in the case of those maimed in warfare (such as the Guinea Pigs, the early plastic surgery successes during the Second World War in 1939–1945). More usually, the difference at best brings a mark of respect for courage in adversity – 'you are brave' – and, at worst, is associated with inferior social standing.

This is the cultural definition of 'visibly different'. It varies between eras, societies and cultures. Victorian England permitted circus acts involving 'freaks' such as the Elephant Man. Asian communities today view disfigurement as 'fate' or 'karma' and the individual is not expected to do more than bear the burden stoically.

Secondly, there is the personal definition, of the person who has an appearance that leads them to feeling visibly different from those around. The extent of the visible difference may actually be quite minor but they *feel* it is significant. Thus, the individual's appearance may not have strayed beyond what might be perceived as the boundaries of 'normal appearance' but the person may still *feel* visibly different.

On which of these criteria am I therefore visibly different?

There is no question that I am indeed visibly different on the social definition because my scars and asymmetrical face and subdigital hand mark my appearance as beyond the boundaries of 'normal'; but I do not *feel* different ... any more. For most of the time, I forget about 'it' and many of my family and friends do not notice at all (or so they say). I think Flat Stanley was right: 'when you get used to it', it can be quite enjoyable. I know that sometimes I can use my different appearance to advantage, but this was not always so. What I went through in the years after my accident was, in retrospect, the bereavement experience of losing my looks, such very important attributes in today's world (and probably, in yesterday's and tomorrow's too). It was certainly not a straightforward transition because there is no 'grieve-by date'. Time can help the healing process but unfortunately this is not automatic: some people continue to feel different for years ... (see Chapter 16).

This book is focused on and dedicated to helping those who do *feel* different, and to those who are very close to them, such as their parents, relatives, partners and siblings. The aim is to open up the experience and offer guidance to those who work to help people to go through this feeling of being different, even if they can never avoid the cultural tag of 'different'.

How 'cultural norms' come about, why they work to the detriment of those who are visibly different, and how they might be changed, are fascinating subjects in their own right, but they are not the main subject matter of this book. Yet it would be wrong not to point out at the outset just how pervasive the cultural forces are about visible difference; these are forces against which any affected individual has to fight. Not only are these in others' minds but they also enter and dominate the affected person's mind.

These forces can be neatly, if somewhat simplistically, summarized in two equations: 'handsome/pretty = good/valuable' and 'ugly/unattractive = evil/unwanted'. The first equation is asserted by the bombardment of advertising, media and films eulogizing about the crucial importance of 'looking good'; the second is stealthily fed through a diet of stereotypical images in horror stories/movies, cartoons, crime and science fiction all linking unprepossessing personality traits to scarred or hideous appearance (see Chapter 15).

Those who have a significant visible difference, such as the people who have written for this Section, would be at one in wishing an end to these equations, but know that they have to live with them. One professor of plastic surgery recently opined that pantomimes like *Cinderella* ought to carry government health warnings, a thought that while slightly overstated, perhaps does certainly capture the difficulty of changing the imagery in vogue 'n western culture.

It should be noted that much of modern plastic and cosmetic surgery is geared to reshaping people's faces and bodies so that they come within normal limits and, preferably, into the so-called attractive end of 'normal'. Contrary to popular belief, however, such surgery has limitations. Some people even after receiving many operations will never come within the 'norm' as it currently exists.

I do believe that visible disfigurement has become an easier subject to talk about in recent years. There is less of a taboo surrounding it. The very public experiences of men such as Simon Weston, the Falklands War veteran and Niki Lauda, the former racing driver, have certainly increased public understanding about burn injuries, for example.

The number of personal accounts of how it has influenced the lives of those affected is, however, still very small. Lucy Grealy's recent book about her facial surgery and aftermath (Grealy, 1994) has won high praise because it is very accessible to the general reader. Similarly, John Updike's *Self-Consciousness* (Updike, 1990) about his skin condition and Dennis Potter's TV drama, *The Singing Detective*, about psoriasis have raised awareness. None of these are what I would call a 'Poor me/you' account, one that makes the reader feel sorry for the person involved. Instead, they are realistic, touching and direct.

My fire: destroyer and creator

Fire is a stupendously awesome element. I have great reverence for it; it has damaged and devastated me and yet it also sustains and enlightens me. In 1970, at eighteen years old, I was transformed from a handsome (yes...) youth to a visibly very different person whose outlook on life changed from the inside. The fire and its aftermath changed me. I have chosen a few brief snippets to illustrate that transformation.

April 1971: After four months in a burns unit, I am given a mirror for the first time to look at my distorted face: all scabs, scars, veins and non-symmetry. I try to put on a brave face but am reduced to crying in the night. I feel so sad and so sorry for myself.

Summer 1971: I go to a party of old friends; excruciating to see how I am avoided yet blissful to sense that I might still be able to party! An old girl friend embraces me...

October 1971: A month into a new university career, I have not stopped talking to myself, pushing myself on to face the world as I walk around with dark glasses and a black hat pulled down. I am exhausted but desperately cling to the dream of surgery and the hope of finding new friends.

February 1972: An evening of drink with someone new; I find I can befriend and am interesting too. Two days later, I hear my surgeon say 'but you do realize that we can only do so much'... agony.

July 1972: Joyce, the ward's tea lady, always joking, notices a glint in my eye. 'You're in love, aren't you?!!' My face doesn't blush any more but I do inside at how obvious it is.... Only a very short affair but an affair....

January 1973: After about twenty visits to theatre (a word that seems very inappropriate somehow), I realize that I will never rejoin the ranks of the 'normals' – forever an outsider – and someone has written a book about it: Colin Wilson, *The Outsider* (1963) and so has Camus and... I dive into the world of outsider literature; I am not alone!!

June 1973: I decide to arrange a year off from university to rebuild my chin. I am suddenly 'in control' of my surgery, having told my surgeon that I think a pedicle is what I need (not knowing what I was letting myself in for). He seemed amazed; perhaps patients aren't meant to do this....

January 1974: Depths of despair as the pedicle already in situ for five months shows signs of failing. It is my only hope. I pray as I have never done before....

July 1974: I come round from the last pedicle operation and demand a mirror: bruising, yes, but a chin. I sleep with relief. Maybe now I can say goodbye to surgery. My parents arrange a small party for the surgeon and his team. It really does feel like the end or is it the beginning? I feel so grateful to my family.

August 1977: I am in work in London and gradually growing in confidence. I meet a woman who has had so much more to mourn than I do. We find a huge common territory incredibly quickly.

January 1985: Married, and living in Guernsey and teaching in a girls' school, I am asked to 'cover' a class of twelve-year-olds. 'Mr Partridge, what exactly happened to you?' It is another opportunity and I take it gently, just as I have always been open with my sixth-form class. Maybe I can open their minds to the richness of living, as I do, damaged face and all. Their maths lesson is somewhat changed as we explore the meaning of life!

June 1986: I go to watch a cricket Test Match in London. In the tube train, I am stared at most invasively. I try to escape but can only leave the scene feeling horribly disfigured again. I spend the rest of the day feeling self-conscious, as if for the first time. I thought I had 'got over it'. Back in Guernsey, I arrange on the phone to meet a man about a field; his first comment is 'Oh, I never realized you looked like that.'

May 1995: My wife and I are at a school sports day. 'It still really annoys me the way people just think they can inspect you.' I smile.

The experience of visible difference

My idea for the first section of this book was to offer ten people who are all visibly different (using the social definition) the chance of writing about their life experiences and thereby to provide readers with an insight into what it is like to live with disfigurement. I cannot claim to have chosen a representative sample of the population of visibly different people, but, having met and spoken to well over 1000 people in this category over the past five years, I can say that they do give a clear picture of most of the major problems that are faced, and of how the experience is at once devastating and yet also enlivening.

The contributors fall into two groups: those who were born with a disfigurement, and those who acquired a disfigurement at some time in their childhood, adolescence or adulthood. The causes of their disfigurements range from the rare to the relatively common.

I have grouped them in this way because I am often asked whether the experience is 'harder' for those who have a disfigurement from birth compared with those who acquire one. My usual answer is that it is difficult to make generalizations. One thing is for sure; visible difference on the face does leave a lot of people feeling different inside too. They want to be respected for this. It does not help to say, 'We're all the same underneath', we're not: human, yes but the same, no.

I do think there are more similarities than differences between such experiences but the most crucial factors in determining how hard any individual finds it are:

- How stigmatizing is the cause of the disfigurement?
- What quantity and quality of social support does the person have?
- What is his or her level of pre-existing self-confidence?
- Is the underlying personality extrovert or not?

Readers are encouraged to note recurring themes as they study the contributions. They are, I think, deeply moving pieces and I thank all of the contributors most sincerely.

I wrote to them as follows:

> I would like to ask you to contribute a piece of written material (about your disfigurement), not necessarily all in straight prose that expresses your experience, and (possibly) three shorter pieces describing how three other people known to you reacted (a member of your family, a health professional, and another person). In all, I would hope that you could keep your contribution to between 2000 and 2500 words.

The responses were unanimously favourable, but almost all found that getting someone else to write the piece was not that easy. Partly because their close friends had, as one of them commented, 'never noticed that I was disfigured'. I have edited all their accounts with a light pen. One contribution is a press feature.

The first piece, however, does not really fit into either the congenital or the acquired camp, but appeared in a national newspaper at the time of writing this chapter. It concerns the loss of a tooth (Lambert, 1995).

In the tooth of a crisis

My front tooth broke off yesterday in the middle of breakfast. I felt it snap. I was just biting into a piece of toast when suddenly there was a strange void. I looked down and saw the tooth nestling like a large crumb in my toast. While my tongue explored the crater it had left behind, my mind raced through the implications.

Fortunately I had no reason to venture out in public until today, when I was booked to do an interview in the afternoon that could not be cancelled. I had 36 hours to solve the problem. By five to eight I was on the phone to my dentist. By a miracle someone was there – someone with a warm, comforting voice who understood the gravity of the case and assured me it would be a small matter to remedy it. 'Come to the surgery any time between 9.30 a.m. and 5.30 p.m. No appointment needed. You count as an emergency.'

I picked up the tooth and took it carefully through to the bathroom. I risked examining the damage in the mirror. A snaggle-toothed, medieval peasant stared back. In the brief second it had taken me to bite, all the advantages conferred by contact lenses and hair colour had been rendered null and void. I was grotesque, fit for the brush of Hieronymus Bosch or a Dutch painting of the 'drunken peasants making merry' genre.

'Does it hurt?' my partner asked as I returned, stricken, from the mirror.

'Hurt? No it doesn't hurt, not in ver least,' I said, discovering a new tendency for 'th' to sound like 'v'.

'That's all right then. Lucky.'

'Lucky? Vis is a dental emergency. I have loft a front toot.'

He turned away and suppressed a snigger. 'Yes, you have, haven't you?' Pause. 'Poor old you.'

I don't remember him ever calling me 'old' before.

An hour later, muffled up to the chin and with a hat pulled low over my eyes, I set out and discovered that on the streets, in public, I had become a changed character. Instead of greeting the street-cleaners, I shuffled past, head bent into my scarf. I didn't risk buying from my usual newspaper seller in case she engaged me in conversation. I had taken on the surly incommunicativeness of the, um, physically challenged.

As I booked my ticket to East Croydon (that's how far you have to travel to find an NHS dentist) the ticket seller demanded the wrong money. I did not allow myself to argue. At Victoria station, rather than accost the nearest figure in BR uniform and demand to know from which platform the next East Croydon train would leave, I meekly scanned the departures board and worked it out for myself.

Miserable, guilty and down in the mouth, I sat on the train immersed in the newspaper. Not for me the winsome game of peep-bo with the adorable toddler opposite. ('Only two-and-a-half? Gosh, he's amazing isn't he?') Today I am Ms Misogynist; stay away from me.

Thank God! East Croydon! I pushed through the crowd and headed doggedly for the dentist, dreading the waiting room. There was only one other person there: a tramp, muffled up against the cold, with a raw, battered face and – ye gods! – a missing front tooth. I looked at him. 'Fnap!' I said.

'Yer wot, Miffuf?' he answered.

My usual dentist was not in. No matter. Any dentist would have done. I followed the receptionist to a small cubicle. A young man with acne (oh, poor him, I found myself thinking, uncharacteristically) greeted me. 'Hi there, hello. Come in. Have I seen you before? Cold enough for you is it?'

I smiled wanly.

'What seems to be the matter?'

The wind whistled through the Cheddar Gorge in the middle of my smile, and he was asking me what was the matter. I bared my lips in a snarl. 'Ah yes. Got the tooth? Right. Won't be a tick.'

The chair was wound down until I was horizontal. Dear me, that acne was bad. He wedged cotton wool between my upper lip and popped the rogue tooth in and out a few times. The dental nurse had prepared an adhesive which he wound round the tooth before jamming it into the gap and propping it there hard against his finger. While he counted to a hundred he crooned to himself: toodly-oo-dee-oo.

Tiddly-om-pom-dee. Pom, I thought. Tiddly-om-pom-*pom*. After a couple of minutes it was set. Miraculous, these new dental fixatives.

'Try not to chew on it today.'

'Thank you,' I said, 'Gosh, that feels marvellous! Thank you.' Suppressing the desire to recommend an awfully good lotion for acne, I made my way out.

'That'll be £5.28,' said the receptionist. I beamed.

'Cheap at the price.'

The moral, if you like, of this story is how pitifully little it takes to shake one's confidence. A tooth falls out – one tiny square of bone and enamel – and I deflate like a balloon. What a fool I must look normally, striding along the streets, head up, eyes front, coat swinging, heels clicking, insufferably pleased with the world!

There must be an ascending scale of humiliation, starting with conjunctivitis, a black eye, a broken leg, right up to... what? Amputation? Paralysis? How do people whose faces have been badly burnt or scarred in an accident muster the courage to venture out each day?

(Reproduced with permission from *The Independent*)

References

Brown, J. (1968). *Flat Stanley*. London: Methuen.

Goffman, E. (1963). Stigma: *Notes on the Management of Spoiled Indentity*. London: Penguin.

Grealy, L. (1994). *Autobiography of a face*. New York: Houghton Mifflin.

Lambert, A. (1995). In the tooth of a crisis. *The Independent*, 11 January, p. 19.

Partridge, J. (1990). *Changing faces*. London: Penguin.

Updike, J. (1990). *Self-Consciousness*. London: Penguin.

Wilson, C. (1963). *The Outsider*. London: Pan Books.

Part One

Congenital Disfigurement

Chapter 2

Maureen Williams

> Maureen is a primary school teacher in Yorkshire. She was born with a large port wine stain that covers most of one side of her face. She is now over fifty and lives with her husband and daughter.

I was born near Liverpool in October 1943, a 'war baby', a normal healthy baby except that the right half of my face was a bright livid red. It must have been a shock for my mum seeing me for the first time but she says she was upset for my sake, besides there was a war going on. My dad was away in the army, the Royal Engineers, and I had a brother Stephen, two years old, waiting at home and my sister Cathryn was to follow me into the world just fifteen months later, so there was plenty to occupy my mum's thoughts. Life then wasn't easy anyway.

It must have caused a bit of an upset in the family though because my mum's parents, grandma and granddad Sedgwick, came over from Mosborough (outside Sheffield) to see their latest grandchild and apparently said, 'We'll have to do something about that!'

Later, when I was a bit older, I was taken to our GP. He didn't think anything could be done but promised to ask around. My Sedgwick grandparents were asking around too, and that's how I came to see a consultant called Mr V.

Isn't it funny how our memories go? When asking the people involved like my mum, dad, my auntie Jose, how little they remember of the details. So the exact age that I paid my first visit to Mr V. the dermatologist (if that was his title?) is unknown, but we think I must have been three or four years old. Mr V. had learnt about a treatment being used in Germany; 'liquid X-ray' my mum called it. Auntie Jose says that it smelt like pear drops and it was supposed to break up the birthmark and disguise it. My grandparents paid for the treatment (two guineas a time, Auntie Jose thinks). I would go to Mr V.'s house with granddad and Jose in the car. Waiting in the room downstairs was a delight. He had a table with puzzles on, the ones where you have to get the ball bearing to a certain place.

Upstairs, Mr V., a tall gentleman, would put 'the stuff' on my birthmark. Later, back at grandmas, this would be wiped off with ether. I can still remember the strong smell of it. During this time I lived with my grandparents to be near Mr V. in Sheffield. I loved them very much, they were wonderful to me and for me. I stayed there, cosseted, until it was time to start school at five or six. My treatment was transferred to a hospital in Liverpool and presumably put onto the National Health. Mr V. himself came over to Liverpool to explain my course of treatment. I returned home to a very different world. Instead of being an only one I was now one of five children. Besides Stephen, me and Cathryn, there was now John and Bridget; Angela, Mary, Josephine, Joseph, Andrew and Thomas were to follow over the next fifteen years.

School was a very strange environment and that's when I first experienced or remember experiencing, being picked on and being bullied because of my face. Until I went to school, I had not felt hurt by having a birthmark; different, yes, getting a lot of attention, yes, and that was nice, but being picked on in a nasty way, that was a shock. I remember two older girls persistently seeking me out in the playground; I know I dreaded it but *what* they did exactly is blocked off in my mind. However, the longer I was at school the more I became known and the more the other children got used to me.

There was another boy, Richard, who was quite deformed and very clever, and other children who were very poor and couldn't afford shoes, so we were all maybe oddballs in some ways. By the time I was in the juniors, I was established – a brother above me, younger sisters and brothers below me – we Price children were well known! I remember being very happy and having lots of friends. I had a decent brain and some artistic ability, so my work was praised and my self-esteem nurtured.

If in school or at home I felt safe, the space in between was a threat. We lived at the bottom of what, to me, seemed a very long road with a rise in the middle. At the bottom end where we lived I knew the people, we played out in the street there, the children next door went to the same school; it was our territory, but, in the middle, that was where, it seemed to me, a lot of older, strange children lived. They went to a different school and they called us names. My sister Cathryn recalls that they shouted 'Rudolph the red-nosed reindeer' after me and she shouted back, 'Don't you call my sister names.' If I was alone, I often went the long way round to and from school to avoid walking through this 'No man's land'. It was at school too that I first had my photo taken, or the only photo of me as a young girl we've got dates from that time. My mum says I hid in the corner when the camera came out.

From junior school, I went on to a convent school in the centre of Liverpool and never looked back. I felt completely at home and valued there. I can't remember an awkward time of getting to know people. The nuns and lay teachers were fair and good. We were part of a happy community. A year later, my sister Cathryn joined me.

I should have mentioned that during my infant school days and early junior days my treatment continued. I can't remember how frequently I went to the hospital but I can remember standing at the bus stop outside school waiting to go for an appointment. I must have been eight or nine years old and been allowed to go by myself; but the treatment wasn't working. Areas of red on my face had faded slightly but other areas were browning. My dad says that the treatment was beginning to damage the skin, so it was stopped. The dream I had of my birthmark disappearing by the time I reached my teens was not going to come true.

The older I became, the more self-conscious I became about my face. I didn't like getting on the bus that took me to and from school. I always tried to sit with my birthmark side to the window away from the other passengers. I dreaded getting off the bus and walking down the aisle facing everyone. I don't know whether it was this fear of facing people that made me deliberately say to myself that, although I hated it so much, it was something I must get used to. I had to do something to harden myself to peoples' staring, so I joined the dramatic society at school. It was run by Sister Therese, a lady we all admired. At least once a year we put on a play for the rest of the school and evening performances for parents and friends. I always took a part, not a leading one, but I was there on the stage, even if only as the third murderer in *Macbeth* or a butler in *Pride and Prejudice*. Sister Therese taught me to speak clearly and well, and to appear confident in front of others, even if I really felt like hiding away.

From the age of about fourteen years, I started to wear glasses; not liking them at first, I tried to struggle on without them. I was reprimanded by the optician who said I could do more damage by not wearing them, so mum and dad bought me a more fashionable pair and I've been happy to wear them ever since. I think I hide behind them a bit (like armour).

When I was in the fifth form, aged fifteen to sixteen years old, the specialist at the hospital arranged for me to make a promised visit to Max Factor in London to learn to apply make-up. Myself and two best friends went down to London for the day and, whilst I learnt the basics of applying foundation, powder, eye make-up etc., they went round the shops. From then on, Max Factor 'Panstick' became my best friend. I came home a different person; I thought I looked like 'a million dollars'. I brought a new coat, I still remember it, creamy white with big pearl buttons and had my photo taken in a studio (mum and dad still have that photo in the family album).

Since that day, I have always worn make-up for work and my social life. With the family and on holiday, especially abroad, I don't wear make-up. I feel I am two different people: my made-up self and my natural self. I remember after returning from London, the geography teacher at school, a nun, saying that she thought I should wear it when I started work, especially if I intended working with children and being a teacher. She felt that I might be at a disadvantage if my birthmark was not covered.

From school I went on to college and I really took off. I was away from home. I felt attractive and for the first time I had boyfriends. People who met me made-up didn't ask questions so I never told them about my face. (Maybe they guessed but if so they never said anything.) I met Richard, my husband, while I was at college and he was at university. After going out with him for some time I became more anxious that he should know the truth, the terrible truth as I saw it at the time. I was very frightened to tell him in case it changed our relationship – in case what he was going to find out made him alter his feelings about me. Looking back I see how silly I was, how I made the whole thing more 'dramatic' than it really was.

I remember that evening vividly. We were meeting to go out into town. We walked down to the bus stop and all the time I was trying to think of the right words to tell him. I kept saying I had something important to say, something serious about me but I couldn't get the word 'birthmark' out. It wasn't until we were sitting on the bus that I came out with it. I'm smiling now because I can remember what he said. He had guessed that my make-up covered some skin disfigurement but he was relieved because he had thought my serious tone and the something important was life-threatening like cancer; what an anticlimax. I had worked myself into a state and made him very worried for something that to him was not a big issue.

Isn't that how it is to the people who know us and really care for us? Our disfigurement is not an issue. We ourselves can make it into a barrier. We ourselves can make it come between us and our dealings with others.

When I think about my birthmark, which is not very often, thank goodness, I see how important my family and my upbringing have been in giving me confidence and strength to go through life, which, at times, when I am in deep despair, does seem very difficult. Writing this has made me think deeply about it more than I have ever done for a long time. From the little girl who prayed that when she woke up in the morning she might look in the mirror and see a face without an ugly red mark, I have become a woman of fifty years old who still hopes for a miracle but in reality knows that I am as I am.

I had a big party when I was fifty; I felt it was a landmark. I never thought I would get this far. As I said, I can have terrible black despairs when to go to sleep and never wake up seems desirable, but, I suppose the older we get the more at ease we become with ourselves.

I have been extremely lucky to have a wonderful family and a wonderful husband just right for me. I have a daughter who is very beautiful and that gives me great joy. It took me a long time to pluck up courage to have a family – thinking that what had happened to me might happen to her – but there were no flaws and that was an immense relief.

I do worry about getting older; it will be a lot harder to disguise my birthmark if I want to. I do worry about going out into Doncaster, where I live, and meeting someone who only knows me wearing make-up. However I do have the confidence to stand up and speak in areas where I feel competent, for example, as a teacher. I am quite willing to stand up in front of an audience and express my views/feelings (as long as I have my notes ready). Being with new people for the first time, I can feel awkward until I get to know them. Once I feel I know them and they know me I can relax and be myself.

The feeling is always there though, that you are different (apart from others). I think you will always feel different because you are different. You are different because you look different. You look different because of that disfigurement which you can't change. Because of that you have a whole area of experience that only others who are disfigured as you are can share; but that does not stop you having all the same feelings as others, the same emotions, likes and dislikes, responsibilities and enjoyments. You have the same entitlements in life and that life might bring more trials but lots of joys too; perhaps it makes you stronger!

By her sister

My parents treated Maureen no differently from the rest of their children, so we grew up doing the same. I can't remember paying much attention to Maureen's birthmark but I must have asked Mum about it once and she just replied that Maureen was born with it and nothing more was said. We never discussed her birthmark. There didn't seem any need. I did think it was rough that she had one but I didn't feel sorry for her because she didn't seem to feel sorry for herself. It seems to me that Mum and Dad and Maureen set the example of not paying too much attention to it and the rest of us just followed suit.

Maureen always had plenty of friends. She always attracted people who enjoyed life. At college she was in with a lively crowd.

Maureen applied her make-up very skilfully and took a lot of care with her appearance. She has good dress sense and she made the most of what she had; she had very dark glossy hair and always looked good when she went out.

By a friend

I first encountered Maureen about fifteen years ago, when her daughter started reception class in the school in which I teach. I remember at the time fleetingly noticing that one of the mums was extremely well made-up, but, obviously, at the time more attention was paid to the daughter – quite a character in her own right. (Maureen is still known ten years later as 'Nerys's mum' amongst the staff at my school!) However, at the time, I only noticed the make-up, immaculate in a catchment area where the usual female above shoulder adornment includes tattoos and love bites!

Just over ten years ago, we moved to our present home, next door to Maureen and her family. At first, as with most new neighbours, we were merely nodding acquaintances. I can clearly remember the first time I saw her bare face. Maureen obviously felt at ease; I did not, and was ashamed of myself for not being.

Since that first occasion, I have seen her both with and without make-up, and can now honestly say that neither face bothers me, apart from sometimes, when we go out and Maureen is immaculately made-up, I feel a bit of a slob for not making any effort.

I do not know, and cannot begin to imagine, the prejudice, discrimination and sheer ignorance that Maureen has had to overcome. Since I have got to know her, and value her friendship, she has always appeared to me to be outgoing, totally confident, and brutally honest. I do not know if these characteristics are in spite of, or because of, her birthmark. I only wish I had half of her confidence!

I have found this exercise extremely hard, to cast my mind back to when I was 'bothered' by Maureen's birthmark. Perhaps it is a sign of my own maturity that I see her only as a person whom I like, not as a person with a birthmark. The most recent example of this is when we arranged, at very short notice, to go out for a meal. I said 'Five minutes.' Maureen said, 'Thirty.' I said, 'Why?' Maureen said, 'I have to put my face on.' I said 'What for, you're fine as you are.' And she is.

Chapter 3

Alan Chapple

Alan is a teacher living in Bristol with degrees in psychology and physics. He was born with a bilateral cleft lip and palate.

I was born in Oxfordshire in May 1957. At that time my parents were resident at RAF Gaydon in Warwickshire. Apart from one thing, we would have been a normal young family growing up in times of increasing prosperity. The difference was that I was born with a hare lip and cleft palate. This was a distorting influence on me and my family from the start. The marital strain imposed by my disfigurement coupled with the frequent journeys to hospital for operations and check-ups throughout my early childhood meant that my family was enduring a far from normal time.

For myself, this family disruption had an isolating effect on me. My experiences took place largely in a vacuum, as I was unable to communicate with my parents for fear of rekindling emotions that were just held in check. The early years were filled with fear, pain and terror.

When I was aged four we moved to North Africa, where life seemed brighter (it was, on the Tropic of Cancer, with the sun directly overhead for most of the hours!), and I learnt rapidly, having space to explore, new friends, and a natural environment. The early unease seemed to fade; family life had meaning again.

Returning to England three years later seemed to be a retrograde step, as I had to unlearn much that I had learned, such as climbing trees, the metric system, writing with my left hand, and taking the initiative wherever possible. There was an early conflict between discipline and freedom. I knew that I was different and was frequently singled out as such, but, according to my teachers and my parents, I was supposed to be the same, and expected to conform to contradictory rules and regulations that were supposedly 'for my own good'. In retrospect, I think my natural exuberance, which was so vital in coping with my disfigurement, was blighted.

My adolescence was a confusing business. I was extremely intelligent, but my physical form was frail. Bullying came in many forms and I very rarely came out on top. From the outset the fear was of 'having my face smashed in', which is how the gang always functioned. They always had safety in numbers, and with veiled threats and taunts, they kept me in perpetual fear. I did have friends but they were often unusual themselves, and usually, though not always, very intelligent.

When my sexuality stirred, I was curious, but as I was heavily repressed and 'told what to do', I came up against a dilemma. No-one could tell me 'what to do' in this case, and so I didn't know how to express my instincts effectively. The result was young lust. I had grown so used to my face being rejected that I couldn't imagine anyone being interested. When, at eighteen, I did find someone who took an interest in me, my sexuality exploded, not into the wonderful world of pleasure and love I yearned for, but almost into insanity. My inner confusions and doubts arose from a deep fear of rejection. My need for security expressed itself as possessiveness to a frightening degree.

Since that time, my life had been more troughs than peaks. Looking at it, I see myself trapped in an enveloping web of rules and regulations, prescriptions and restrictions which other people have decided to impose on me. I have a particularly poor view of the local authority, the bank manager and the health care system all of whom I feel have failed to help me. Instead I feel my brain has been abused by the effects of drugs I was prescribed and I am still a prisoner of the infernal system of state hand-outs upon which I frustratingly depend.

My lack of a permanent job and partner is compounded frequently by infuriating incidents. For example, I recently cycled through the dirt and pollution of Bristol to do a day's supply work in a local junior school. Somehow, I managed to get through the day, and felt better for doing it. The trouble was that having no bank account meant that I couldn't be paid! I have now sorted that one out.

I also look back on the tragedy of my girlfriend's death in 1987 and a car accident in 1989 as sources of pain that I am still trying to resolve. I feel as if both these events caused me to lose my sense of purpose and self-reliance. In early 1988, when I went through every emotion that man can summon, I returned to a difficult home situation. Now, back in isolation after years of failure, I find myself with a second degree in psychology, looking back. What are the reasons? Perhaps I have been a self, that became over self-obsessed due to being a 'done-to' for too long, and a lot has crept up behind me. The test is to overcome my fear. Because I have been led to expect rejection, I have now become almost indifferent to it.

I recently asked a very attractive young lady and friend in our guitar group if she would accompany me to a workshop and concert at the Bristol Music Club, Clifton. To my surprise and delight, she accepted, and I put aside my anger, and did some preparation. Two days later, the isolation was getting worse. There was a crippling depression descending upon me, but, three days on, our group met at the local grammar school and we spent a wonderful evening together. I felt less separate, more connected. A future has to be shaped, in order that the isolation will never recur. But it is so difficult when your mind set is negative.

And beyond....

Midlife is often a time of searching for new meanings. I am lucky enough to have known love, and was blessed with plenty of intelligence, but not always wisdom! So, at thirty-seven, I have found myself painfully thrown back on my own resources and made aware of my physical limitations. My face has been the source of so much anguish and yet, in happy times, it has smiled and laughed as freely as any!

In troubled times, I believe that it is essential (whatever the 'normals' try to tell you) to be happy and find your own unique purpose in life. There is no-one else quite the same, and no matter how hard you try, you just won't fit into a box forever.... That is, if you want to live!

Chapter 4

Katherine Lacy

> Katherine Lacy has a hereditary skin condition called neuro-
> fibromatosis. She is in her fifties, and has specialized in health
> education/health promotion. She is a counsellor and self-
> development trainer who lives in Kent.

I have a hereditary skin condition called neurofibromatosis (Nf) or von
Recklinghausen's disease after the German Physicist (1833–1910) who first
described it. It consists of many benign noncancerous tumours caused by an
overgrowth of the cells surrounding the nerves. 'Lumps and bumps', you
could call them. When they first emerge, I may get a tingling sensation, but,
apart from this, they are not painful unless I hit them or they rub and bleed.

I was first aware of being 'different' when at the age of six, I went into a
children's hospital for an operation on my face. I remember being told
something about the enamel on my teeth not forming properly. This
meant that my back teeth and adult molars had to be cut out from the
jaw. Explanations to small children were not as common as they are
today. I recall two 'doctors', one a 'specialist', an elderly, austere man,
who I found very intimidating. Mr S. was younger, and much more gentle
and I trusted him.

When it came to having the 'pre-med' I was given it crushed up in a
spoonful of jam. I did not like jam and refused to take it. On being force
fed, I was promptly sick and they had to start all over again. My Nanny,
who was with me for the whole of my stay in hospital, apart from the nights,
was sent out of the room. Mr H. came in to make me take the medicine. He
found me quite hysterical and was not best pleased when I called him the
very worst thing that I could think of: 'You devil.' This must have been the
first time he had met a challenge for many years. He was very angry.
Although I can't remember what he said, I do remember what he did. He
lifted up my nightie and slapped me hard on the thigh. I thought he was
going to kill me. (I'll bet he felt like it too!) I looked at the red imprint of his
hand on my flesh. It was the only time I had ever been hit in my life.

After the operation, what was prominent in my mind was that it was
September and that my birthday was in October. I *had* to be home for

my birthday. Each day I would ask my Nanny 'What month is it?' She knew my feelings about being home for my birthday but was not party to the confidences of the staff as to when I was likely to be discharged. In answer to my question she always answered 'September' and I was satisfied. One morning however, when I asked my usual question, as she replied 'September', a nurse who had just come into the room replied 'October'. A frisson went through me. In three days I was well enough to go home. The nurses, my mother told me later, had never seen anyone make such a speedy recovery.

I also had two quite large neurofibromata: one on my upper right arm, the other on my left chest. I don't know why they didn't remove them when I was in the hospital because I had pointed them out to the doctors and nurses, asking them to take them away too; but no-one listened to a six-year-old girl.

These two 'spots' were a source of fascination and fear to children at school. They often wouldn't play with me. Most of my school years were spent wandering alone around the playground. The mothers of the children had told them to keep away from me in case it was 'something nasty' and 'catching'. My attempts to reassure that it wasn't, didn't carry weight. 'You would say that, wouldn't you?' I finally persuaded my parents to let me have the spots taken off, but the operation was not very successful. The stitches broke and left large disfiguring scars, which were not dealt with until I was much older.

It was not just schoolchildren who were a pain in my life. Some of the teachers too betrayed how much they associated 'ill looks' with 'ill nature'. I wasn't allowed to forget. I remember many incidents to this day; here are three:

In my class, some of the children's books had been scribbled over in red crayon. Every child in the class was asked if they had done it. No-one owned up. Two girls were asked a second time. One of them was me. Even at that date, I was nine, I knew about 'facial discrimination'. I said to the teacher, 'You only asked Deborah and me again because we are the two ugliest in the class, and it's not me!' In the summer of 1993, I came in touch with that teacher again at a school reunion. It took a long time before I could bring myself to go and say, 'How do you do?' Sadly I never said, 'You know I never did scribble on those books.' I was trying to convince myself that she wouldn't have remembered anyway. I was surprised at how strongly my sense of injustice and anger had come back that afternoon.

Eating sweets was not allowed in class. I was once accused of this. The proof, when I denied it, was that the teacher could see the lump in my cheek where it was lodged. I responded with, 'Well, I'm not then – look,' and opened my mouth wide to prove my innocence. I was then in trouble for being rude!

In my last term at school, the head teacher decided to produce a nativity play. I had set my heart on playing Melchior, the most mysterious of the Three Wise Men. I was given the part of Herod!

Over the years I have probably had about 700 neurofibromata removed. Now, unless they are very visible on my face or likely to get hit and damaged, I've decided not to have any more removed. Plastic surgery can only go so far. I have been pleased with what I have had done, but do not want to take the risk of worse scars or facial paralysis. David Matthews, an eminent plastic surgeon, who did a number of the operations, made a big impression on me, when he said not to look for plastic surgery to provide the answers. A lot depended on my developing my talents and personality.

Somewhere around my mid-twenties, I knew I wanted to have a fulfilling career. This called for further education, and at least a degree. I did not have the confidence to leave my job and go to university, so I decided that a degree at evening classes was the best path of action and went to what was then the Central London Polytechnic. I spent four-and-a-half years going for two nights a week to evening classes. This was on top of a full-time job. During evenings and weekends, when not at college, I would spend up to two hours a day studying. The hard work paid off and I gained an upper second honours degree. My then boss, who had no degree, was very dismissive and told me in a staff meeting that the only degree worth getting was a 'first'. Later, I obtained an MSc in health education. When asked if I was going to do a PhD too, I laughed and said I didn't need to be 'Dr Lacy' (though thinking it over now, it might be rather fun!). Education has done much to bolster my self-esteem and confidence.

Another challenge that I gave myself was to do a massage course. My body was covered in hundreds of neurofibromata. Stripping off in front of others in a mixed group and being massaged with oil was, on the first day, something of a shock. However, the initial embarrassment went almost immediately and I enjoyed both having the massage done to me and doing it. For some of the others, having to massage me was pretty scary. One student said helplessly to the tutor 'What am I supposed to do with *that*?' He said briskly to treat me like any one else and to check out what I did and didn't like.

What of my family? My father, who dabbled in Christian Science for a while, thought faith healing might help. 'How? What will they do?', I asked. He said they might invite me to think 'better thoughts'. So *that's* what it was all about. God's punishment for being bad, either in this life or a previous one. I was the result of the wrath of God to the third and fourth generation. I spent some time trying to work out which generation I was and whether any children I had would also be punished in a similar way. I decided not to take that risk.

My mother was totally mystified about where it had come from. *Her* family had always been known for their beautiful skin. I felt like a leper. For a while, I felt great affiliation with Charlotte Mew's *The Changeling* and was convinced I was just that: a changeling.

My Nanny, who stayed with us until she died, was an unfailing support, but never a pitier. She encouraged a sturdy approach in me and not to hide away. This was, not always easy. I was very bitter for many years.

Some years ago, I took part in a research project on Nf at Guy's Hospital. They did not X-ray my brain, but I was given to understand that some people with Nf have abnormal brain patterns.

I didn't know about LINK (the self help group, Let's Increase Knowledge about Neurofibromatosis). When I did, I was interested to discover that many of the things that I had known to be true about myself were part of the diagnosis of Nf: shorter than the other members of the family; slightly larger head; problems with co-ordination (I was lousy at games, was always last to be picked in any teams and was greeted with groans, when left over at the end and allocated to one team or the other: 'Now we'll lose!'); appalling handwriting ('poor, careless and illegible' was the end of term report from the writing teacher); and a major difficulty with maths.

What have I found most irritating about my 'condition'? Probably more than the condition itself is the reactions I get from people who are probably well-intentioned but have almost no tact. I think I have developed some very assertive responses over the years! Some of the more common are:

- Strangers who think they have the right to ask what it is: 'I hope you don't mind my asking, but...? My answer can vary from 'I do mind' to a full (if slightly sarcastic) account of medical detail.
- Loud comments for all and sundry to hear. I now refuse to crawl humiliatingly out of the situation but try to isolate the perpetrator.
- A woman on the bus travelling to work saying, 'Your mother played with frogs when she was having you.' This folklore mythology is less heard today but other misconceptions have taken its place. My usual response is to explain that the cause of Nf has yet to be established but frogs have been ruled out. I have also thought how amusing it would have been to have told her I was the Frog Princess and blown her a kiss!
- Well-intentioned individuals recommending faith healers who 'Have wonderful success with warts.' I usually feign listening while wondering whether the faith healer could do much about tactlessness.
- People who give me pitying looks, as if I was terminally ill. These are usually best dealt with with a warm smile.
- Being described as 'very brave and courageous'; if done to my face, I now accept the compliment and change the subject!

There are some things that I won't do: wear short sleeves, or a normal bathing suit. The last time I was on a beach was on a wonderful Caribbean holiday. At one point I was on my own, when a little boy of about four years came up and asked what those lumps were on my hand. I attempted to ignore him but he was quite persistent. Not knowing how you explain a genetic condition to a small, strange child, I lost my cool and stood up and flapped my arms at him and said, 'Go away!' Scaring small children is not something I want to do. I fear I may have reinforced the 'monster image' in his mind. I hope not. Today, I would probably invite him to come and have a look, give a simple explanation and reassure him that they are not painful and that he wouldn't catch them off me.

Today, I feel that my skin is not a deterrent to leading a full exciting life. It is important to show that I am not as bad as I look. I want to help to destroy the stereotype of fairy stories, as 'baddies' in films, books and comics. Whilst not pretending that it is always easy, the pain of *not* living life to the full is far more painful. Although I know that I am likely to go on developing more neurofibromata as I get older, along with a small risk of them becoming cancerous, I am not prepared for that to put my life on 'hold'. There are too many exciting things to do.

Joining Changing Faces has been the first time that my Nf has had a positive outcome. Participants on courses know that I have 'been there' and am talking from a standpoint of tackling difficult situations. I don't just use the textbook theory. I can empathize with the problems, pass on the lessons I have learned, but, most of all, I can encourage people to look to the bright side!

By her elder sister

Katherine (or Monica as we call her) was born with a 'naevus' on her arm and her chest. Because she was a lot younger than my sister and me, and needed a good deal of medical care, she was given extra from the family rations during the war. Being as greedy as most children, we rather resented this.

Our Nanny, who had come to us at my birth, was devoted to Monica's welfare, perhaps not always to her benefit. During air raids, when we sat in the cellar listening to the crashes of the guns and sometimes bombs, Nanny held Monica tightly on her lap, clutching her hand at each bang. Not very reassuring to a small child[1]. When Monica was in her teens I talked to Nanny about what I saw as her possessiveness, asking if she could let Monica go, but Nanny just cried.

As I grew older and started going out and eventually left home, I saw a good deal less of my youngest sister, and only vaguely noticed that the bumps on her body were spreading, and, as she grew up I found it too painful to consider seriously what she must be going through. I found it a particularly horrifying experience visiting her in hospital on one occasion when she had them all removed[2], and I knew that this was only one of several occasions.

For a long time I thought Monica was very angry; who wouldn't have been in her situation? Later, she began to alter the direction of her life. In recent years she has calmed; her new job has given her purpose and self-confidence. She has turned something negative into something very positive.

Notes: Katherine Lacy

[1]I found it very reassuring and never remember being afraid.
[2]Only the worst 300!

By a friend

I first met Kathy almost ten years ago. I had just completed a postgraduate diploma in health education, having made a career change from teaching, and wanted to find some part-time work. I had written to all of my local health promotion units. Kathy was the only one to respond, inviting me to make an appointment to meet her. I have no memory of noticing Kathy's skin condition, I only have a memory of meeting a lively, enthusiastic person who convinced me that I had made a good change of career, and offered me some part-time work.

I feel this is due in part to Kathy's happy personality, determination, strength of character and enthusiasm for life. She takes a pride in her appearance, her hair is well cut, she dresses well and uses make-up skilfully. I feel that Kathy's thirst for advancement and learning has also played a part in developing her confidence to cope in such a positive way. Despite her own problem she has the amazing ability to put people at their ease and indicate real interest in their problems and helping them to overcome them.

I have, however, on occasion seen Kathy depressed and unhappy and it is at that time when you are most aware of her skin condition. As I have come to know Kathy better we have talked about her feelings and of experiences she has had when strangers have asked pointed questions or she has had to cope with whispers and stares. I have great admiration for her and the way she has coped.

Chapter 5

Marc C. Crank

Marc is a postgraduate classics student at the University of Wales. He has a form of neurofibromatosis. He and his girlfriend have just become engaged.

I was born a healthy looking baby but by the age of eighteen months I had started to show signs of what turned out to be a congenital condition, neurofibromatosis. This caused tumours to grow on nerve cells in the right side of my head and face which were to necessitate much surgery later. My surgery started when I was aged three and since then I have undergone a number of craniofacial and cosmetic operations, hopefully to improve both my condition and my appearance.

Now aged twenty-five, I have recently had what is probably my fifty-fourth operation; we lost count after the thirty-sixth. The frequent nature of my hospital stays is at last beginning to abate although I could never envisage a time when there was no longer the prospect of some surgery on the horizon.

The surgery I have undergone has without doubt been most beneficial. We have been told that, without it, I would not be alive today. It has not, however, been without cost. The frequent and often lengthy stays in various hospitals has meant a disrupted school career. The operations have improved my appearance tremendously but these procedures and my complaint combined have left me with much scarring, asymmetry and the loss of my right eye.

The disadvantages I suffer as a result of having lost my right eye are insignificant in comparison with those problems raised by my actually looking different.

Is it possible to lead a 'normal', happy and fulfilled life whilst also being disfigured? Judging by my own life I should say it is so. I had a very happy childhood regardless of the frequent stays in hospital; some hospitals became more like second homes. I achieved well at school and college and I am now in the final year of my degree and looking forward to the possibility of taking a postgraduate degree.

My mother has always insisted that my disfigurement did not make me an inferior person. This has been central to my life. I believe it is imperative that the concept is embraced of being a fully functioning member of society who merely looks different. Without this, the disfigured person cannot carve out their own niche but will be forced to accept that which others place them in.

This is often easier to say than to put into practice. The pain, embarrassment and distress that a disfigured person can feel is not necessarily caused with cruel and malicious intent. The most well intentioned remarks can even be distressing if they come at the wrong time or in the wrong place.

The disfigured person often cannot hide or disguise their 'difference' and must wear it like a badge. All too frequently complete strangers regard the fact that one looks different as a sign that they can walk up to you and demand intimate details about your disfigurement. It seems that they believe they have a right to ask personal questions whether they know you or not.

This is a situation that I have encountered often. Once while visiting the Tower of London, a group of three adults started to stare at me, point and discuss me from the other side of the road. They were so intrigued that they rounded up as many of their friends, relatives and anyone else that was interested, to join their group and continue staring, pointing and discussing me. It was an awkward experience for me but they seemed oblivious that I would be even 'feeling' anything.

At the age of fifteen I had a particularly large operation, which necessitated wearing a bandage that covered a great deal of my head and all of the disfigured parts. The effect of the bandage was quite unexpected; I now looked as though I was the victim of some accident and that the disfigurement was to some extent temporary. I sensed this made a big difference to the way many people treated me. It seemed that to look 'different' was more acceptable if the disfigurement was not permanent and not the result of illness or inheritance.

The liberating effect of the bandage was such that I continued to wear it for seven years, much longer than it was necessary for medical reasons. I continued to have surgery in these seven years which improved my appearance to the extent that I drew more attention with the bandage than I did without it. I still clung on to it for a short while; it was my barrier or 'security blanket' and as such it was hard to let it go. When I did finally stop wearing it, my first few journeys without it were quite traumatic. Once I had again become used to the sensation of wind in my hair and experienced the pleasures of going to a barber. I wondered how ever I had coped for seven years.

Even though my appearance has improved greatly, there are still times when the fact that I do look different is pushed home rather bluntly. In May 1992, I was able to secure the candidature, albeit one that my party have never and could never win, in the local government elections. I was to be the youngest candidate at twenty-three. Because of this, a local paper was interested in writing a piece about me. I was interviewed over the telephone and the reporter asked for photographs so that they could print an article. When this reporter received my pictures his reaction was, 'My God you look ill!' I suggested that his eyes and brain might indeed perceive me as ill but that actually I was quite 'well'. The final format of the article was three lines on some obscure page; the interview was never used, neither were the pictures. I feel very strongly that the decision not to print was due to my appearance. I am of the opinion that the reporter's reaction supports this belief.

There have been so many incidents that I could write pages of anecdotes. However, I feel that this would be negative and would achieve nothing. They can be used to illustrate a point, but to dwell on them is a waste of time. I do not feel that the quality of my life has been diminished by looking different. I genuinely believe that I have gained more as a result of my looks than I have lost by them. I have met some remarkable people who I would not have met if I looked 'normal' and I am extremely lucky that my friends and my fiancée love me for who I am and not for what I look like. How many Helen/Adonis look-alikes can say that confidently?

My looks have shaped me into the person I am today, perhaps giving me greater character, compassion and the vital sense of humour that I may not have otherwise developed. It is not just the actual 'looking different' that has shaped me, but the experiences I have had and the decisions I have had to make. One of the important choices I have had to make was whether to fight for what I really wanted in life or take what society decided I should have. I have my mother to thank for this determination; she has always refused to accept second best for me.

This choice has faced me at almost every stage of my life. In education we had to fight pretty hard for schooling that suited my intelligence and needs, not my looks. With regard to my treatment, the choice becomes more complicated. We have had to struggle to find surgeons that will operate on me. This was a major problem until I was thirteen and first went to Great Ormond Street Hospital for Sick Children.

Once I come under the care of a surgeon, the problem then becomes that they see what they can do, and what they want to do, with one's face which is not always good news. I know what I dislike most about my face and that may not be the most 'abnormal' thing about it. It can be quite a task persuading a surgeon that 'I know the skin on my forehead is scarred but I don't care; what I really want is my ear moving two centimetres!'

It is not always the surgeon who is reluctant. I have made more 'comebacks' than 'The Who'. My postgraduate funding worries would be greatly eased if I had a pound for each time I had said, 'That is it! I don't want any more surgery. Never again!' I am told I usually say this after any particularly painful or problematic operation and it may take a week or more before I change my mind. Not all my operations have been successful; several have been great disappointments. When one has been through quite a lot of pain and discomfort, it is not always easy to stay optimistic and enthusiastic. It can be tempting to say, 'I like me, other people like me, so why bother?'

The decision to have more surgery is because I want to change something about me, not because the world says I should try and look a certain way. The next operation I want may be to make something more comfortable or safer, it is not always a question of improving how I look, rather how I feel. The two are very much linked; there may be some part of me nobody notices but I would *feel* better if it were changed.

There are some things that I cannot change; that I have neurofibromatosis is something that will not change regardless of how I look. This is not something which perturbs me greatly probably because I am not completely certain of the implications, I am not so sure anyone is. I have been told that there may be side-effects such as concentration difficulties and unaccountable fatigue. However, these are 'maybes', so there is no point in worrying about them. They may help to explain the occasional catnap but then so could that tedious lecture. I have enough that I could worry about without including 'maybes'.

Another area in which I have been given conflicting information is genetics. This is a complex subject and differing opinions are inevitable. My condition is usually hereditary but I show none of the standard signs of this and I have been told that my neurofibromatosis is spontaneous. Others have told me that I must have a history of it somewhere in my family. My parents were told that any other children they had may have this complaint. Their decision not to have any more children was not coloured by this so much as by their realization of how much care I would need. They knew that other children without my condition could feel left out because of the attention I would frequently receive.

I have been told that I may pass neurofibromatosis on to my children, but the most recent verdict is that this is unlikely, given the spontaneous nature of my condition. I like the last diagnosis and, as it is the most recent, I shall stick with this. Even if I could pass my complaint on to my children the chance of it manifesting itself in the same way is very unlikely, I am told. My fiancée and I have discussed this matter and we agree that we would like children, regardless. It is the quality of life that is important and I have never wished that I had not been born. In fact, I cannot recall ever wishing I had been born any differently.

Life is only what one makes of it; any situation may be made positive with effort. Being disfigured makes no difference to this. Life can be difficult enough without one giving it a helping hand. Life can be so much easier with help, which is there for almost everybody if they actually look for it. I have been tremendously fortunate to have had the help and support of some very special people: my mother, my surgeon (who I consider a great friend), my general practitioner, friends and now my fiancée. Without these people my life would be so much different.

Chapter 6

John Storry

John was born with a significant malformation of the lower part of his face. Surgery to repair the malformation has spanned a period of thirty years. He now works in the computer industry. His story starts in the 1940s soon after his birth.

I am taken to see a plastic surgeon. His view is that my facial deformities will correct themselves as I get older. He does not explain how and his view is not challenged.

I am at the top of my school class. My father gives me a threepenny-piece as a reward. I will always remember the look on his face. It is a mixture of bewilderment and derision. He cannot equate deformity with intelligence. He is unable to accept my deformity. I feel that he is ashamed of me.

I am out with a friend. We become involved with strangers. They are older. One looks at me, laughs and says to his friend, 'What's this?'

After school I travel home by bus. I alight along with other passengers. As the bus starts to move a window on the upper deck slides open. A youth puts his mouth to the window and yells, 'Hi ya flat nose.' All around me look at the window and then at me. If only there was a hole that I could climb into. I am becoming accustomed to comments such as 'flat nose' and 'flat face'. To me, it is normal and I do not challenge it.

I am the cox of the rowing crew which is successful at the Peterborough regatta. A photograph of the triumphant crew appears on the front page of the local newspaper. I am terrified. The article will draw attention to me.

There is a mirror hanging on the wall. I also have a mirror in my hand. I want to see my profile. I stand sideways to the wall and look into the mirror. I am horrified. My nose is completely flat and, together with my upper jaw, is impacted into my face. My lower jaw extends far in front of the rest of my face. My chin recedes. The whole effect is grotesque. I now understand why I encounter the comments, the looks and the indifference. Instantly, I feel mutilated, repulsive, unlovable and humiliated. My self-acceptance evaporates completely.

My relationship with others changes. I now feel awkward and inferior. My mind concentrates only on my disfigurement. I am unable to accept that anyone wants to be with me.

In public, in a shop, on a bus, at work and with friends it is vital to communicate. Communication, negotiation and assertion is via one's face. We do not talk to or through our feet. My face is damaged. I cannot hide my hideousness and my ability to communicate is impaired.

I cannot bear to show anyone my profile. I am too embarrassed and I always turn away. This stays with me, despite improvements to my face. My apparent indifference to others upsets them. It hurts me much more. It is impossible to explain. I cannot make new friends and my existing friends gradually disappear.

I walk away from disputes. Comments attract attention from others. I want to avoid this at all cost. Gradually, I learn how to handle the comments. I anticipate them and I steel myself against them. I erect a barrier around me. It is equivalent to armour plate. Nothing can penetrate and I am safe. Conversely, nothing can escape. My social and emotional development stops. My feelings and my emotions are completely suppressed.

As a member of the sixth form I sit at the head of the table together with a schoolmaster during the lunch break. The rest of the table is occupied by boys from lower forms. I am not familiar with them and I utter few words. There are many days when I say nothing. The boys talk amongst themselves. My feeling of being ill at ease spreads to the schoolmaster but he makes no attempt to involve me in the conversation.

My father asks me if I have done what he asked. I tell him that I haven't and he asks why. I blurt out that I do not have a face like him. 'What is the matter with it?' he sneers. I walk away feeling even more lonely and vulnerable. This is the only time that my father refers to my disfigurement. I cannot recollect any other discussion.

If anything can be done to correct my deformity, which I doubt, I conclude that it will be me who must take the initiative. No-one else appears to care. My environment does not encourage me to talk about my problem. There is no support, guidance or direction of any kind. I am simply an embarrassment to those around me. I conclude that they all consider the problem to be too severe to be addressed.

I walk to the football match with some friends to watch a first-division game. We are near the ground and I am speaking. My voice falters in mid-sentence. It is as if it has lost its confidence. This is another psychological effect of disfigurement. From this moment, group involvement is difficult. Putting my point of view becomes impossible. The confidence is simply not there. I lose interest in the football. For ninety minutes I stare at everyone around me. All have noses, lips and pleasant curves when looking at their profiles. I think of mine and my despondency gets worse. As I get older I become more sensitive to my disfigurement and I withdraw deeper into my shell. Others also become more sensitive. Doors begin to close and my friends become fewer. My disfigurement is too distressing and too ugly to be part of their environment. I sense the resentment of others when I am around.

I have an interview with a major engineering company. The personnel department is a room set high in the main manufacturing plant. There are chairs around the perimeter. Most are occupied. I go to the reception, which is an enclosed cubicle with a sliding door. I ring the bell and the door slides open. The receptionist is a dark-haired girl, perhaps two or three years older than me. She looks at me and, without saying anything, she bursts out laughing. I feel all of the occupants of the room looking at me. I desperately need a hole to get into. The laughter subsides and she puts her hand to her face to suppress the giggles. Finally, she is able to ask me what I want. I remember little of the interview but I am employed as an electrical apprentice.

I learn that my father has finally left us. I am not surprised or upset. I must improve my face and I resolve to return to my home town as soon as possible.

I visit the labour exchange. I have two interviews, two offers and accept the second. Afterwards I wander around the city centre feeling utterly isolated, alone and dejected.

I have become a recluse. I shun public transport. My bicycle is many times more amenable even in the worst of weathers. I write to an aunt requesting a loan to pay for plastic surgery. The response is one sentence in a letter to my mother. 'Does his face worry him?' The psychological effects get worse. It is difficult to stop the mucus produced by my bowel from running down the inside of my leg. Going into a shop is a miserable experience. I have a tacit agreement with my brother: I take the dog for a walk, he does the shopping. One day I am out with him and we come across a girl from work and I say 'hello' to her. Later, I tell my brother that she is attractive. His response is pragmatic. He says resignedly, 'Forget it.' The comments and actions by females are especially hurtful. During a works' gathering at the local hostelry, I kiss an attractive stranger under the mistletoe. I shall not forget the look of horror that spreads across her face when she realizes who has kissed her. A mother uses her arm to prevent me from talking to her daughter. I become inured to the slights by erecting my barrier. These actions reinforce it. I am intelligent and sensitive but I have to accept that I cannot have a deep, satisfying and intimate relationship. I withdraw further into myself. It is the only way to cope. I cannot be loved and I cannot love. I am told that personality is more important than surface appearance. The statement is correct but it overlooks one critical factor. I think it is impossible to develop an attractive personality with a damaged face.

I have an appointment with a plastic surgeon. Immediately, I feel at a disadvantage. The surgeon can see the subject of our discussion. I can only imagine it and it is difficult to refute some of his comments.

My first operation: bone is taken from my hip and grafted on to my face. My hip hurts tremendously for several days and it is some time before I can walk again. My face does not hurt but the bruising is intense. There are bright hues of yellow, brown and crimson. The plaster is removed after two weeks. Technically, the surgeons have done a wonderful job. I can breathe through my nostrils but I am bitterly disappointed at the aesthetic result. I have a bridge but my nose remains flat. I have a problem and I had assumed that the NHS would identify the cause and recommend a series of operations to correct it. I soon learn that my assumption is naive. If I am to make progress, I will have to cajole the surgeon to undertake further surgery.

I take dancing lessons to try and make some social progress. It is a waste. The dance room has mirrored walls. I look at my image and see an utter mess. I cannot concentrate and my progress is zero. For several weeks I go to the local dance hall with a colleague from work. I do not have the confidence or the skill to ask a girl to dance.

I visit my GP. He is perplexed by my case and discusses it with another doctor. My medical records are on his desk and I glance through them. There is a letter from a plastic surgeon whom I had seen recently. I remember the surgeon telling me that my disfigurement was acceptable and that people soon got used to it. His letter to my GP says something very different. The disfigurement is dreadful but there is nothing that can be done to correct it.

I have an appointment with an orthodontist. His secretary is very helpful and I am relaxed. When I enter the consulting room I am surrounded by medical students. The orthodontist asks me if they can listen to what I have to say. I raise no objections, after all, they have to learn. I am asked to explain my problem. Surely they can see for themselves, but I go ahead. My words flow easily and I feel that I explain adequately. Perhaps this is a good omen. A plaster cast is taken of my jaws and the orthodontist explains that he can set back my lower jaw and eliminate the prognathous effect. As I drive home, I feel a huge sense of relief. The operation will not provide a complete solution but I feel that it will offer significant improvement.

I visit the orthodontist again. His news is disappointing. Setting back the lower jaw will not give me an adequate bite. He will have to set it back further than he originally envisaged. It can be done, but it will affect the hinge of my jaw. He warns me that such an operation can be extremely dangerous. I am desperate for any improvement and I tell him to go ahead.

The orthodontist tells me that he has further researched the situation. One of my facial angles is too narrow. He can correct it, but it will mean moving both jaws. The significance does not sink in.

I am taken to the operating theatre at 7.30 a.m. My teeth were capped the previous afternoon. I am wheeled back to the ward around 11.30 a.m. My jaws are wired together and I cannot move them. Blood trickles down my throat and I find it difficult to breathe.

The swelling starts to subside and my spirits lift but it will be several days before I can leave the hospital. I am unable to eat solid food; for the next two months it must be liquidized. The nurses ask why I waited so long to have the operation. Communication within the NHS is not always good and it is only by chance that I came across the orthodontist.

The orthodontist demonstrates what he did to me with the help of a human skull. Setting back the lower jaw was relatively simple. The front of my skull, together with my upper jaw, was detached and moved forward. It is held in place by bone inserts and wire loops around both cheeks. The operation has transformed my profile. My neighbour is astonished. There are no external scars. All of the work has been carried out through my mouth. No wonder it was sore, but I realize that the engineering behind the operation is absolutely superb.

My surgeon attempts to enlarge my nose. There is much bruising but the attempt fails. He tells me that he is experimenting with treated human tissue, called collagen. A fellow surgeon has it implanted in his arm to test for rejection.

My surgeon puts a large mass of collagen into my nose. The bruising, together with the bandages and wire supports, do not have a pleasing effect. It is well into the following year before the healing process is at an end. Two extrusion points finally heal but they leave dark indents in my nose. My nose is enlarged but the columella is well below the nostril line and askew. It does not look attractive.

I am beginning to get desperate. Time is passing by and, although my face has been vastly improved, I am still very unhappy with my amorphous nose, the columella and the lack of curvature around my lips and chin. My surgeon offers a solution but he cannot promise success. He suggests I solicit the view of other surgeons. Getting them together takes months. I see three of them during a boring day at their clinic. After several weeks, none has responded and I write to remind each of them. I see my surgeon and he tells me that none recommend further surgery. After a lengthy discussion he agrees to operate.

The day of the operation. I worry beforehand. Will I lose my sight? What happens if it goes wrong? Will the result be worth the discomfort? I discuss the situation with my surgeon prior to the anaesthetic. If there is insufficient blood supply, he will stop the operation immediately. I am too desperate to care.

The operation is complete and I awake at 3 a.m. I need to visit the bathroom. There is a mirror over the wash basin. I wash my hands and glance apprehensively at the mirror and quickly look away. I did not see the normal swelling or sticking plaster. I look again. My face is longer. I have a chin. My nose looks different. The base of the columella is level with the outer nostrils. I appear to have lost my shadow around the left nostril. The aesthetic improvement is tremendous. I get back into bed and wonder if I have a face at last.

For several weeks I begin to feel like a human being. My mind slowly, so very, very slowly, begins to believe that my face is almost acceptable to others and to me. I begin to feel that I can go anywhere without fear of ridicule. However, it is a slow process. I am in a bookshop. Behind me two girls are talking and giggling. My defence rises and I dare not look in their direction. After all the reconstruction it would be too much if I discover that I am the source of their merriment. I pass them as I leave the shop. They do not look at me. My relief is immense.

At work, a young lady looks at me. My initial reaction is to erect my barrier. I say inwardly, 'Yes, I know I am disfigured, you will get used to it.' However, she continues to look. In the corridor, in the restaurant and at the coffee machine. She has magnificent blond hair and one of the loveliest faces that I have ever seen. After several weeks, I want to talk to her but the difference between her beauty and my perceived ugliness and repulsiveness is too great. The core problem remains and has a powerful influence on my mind. My past experiences are deeply rooted and I know that if I approach her I will become a bumbling idiot. The thought of rejection is too strong and I am unable to approach her or speak to her. My apparent indifference offends her. I simply feel so damnably wretched.

It is three months since my operation. I enter a building society. I want to change my account. The cashier is not familiar with my requirements. She apologizes for the delay and I tell her that I am not in a hurry. She is attractive and friendly and there is some conversation between us. She completes the transaction and I leave thinking that she has enjoyed our brief contact.

I begin to feel uncomfortable. It is several moments before realization dawns. I also enjoyed the contact. I did not need my barrier. I was an equal. I contributed to the conversation. It was a brief friendship but I found it satisfying and fulfilling. I have experienced the wonders and delight of a relationship for the first time. I have experienced life. I am a human being at last. I can at last direct my life. I can choose, I can select. I am not restricted by the hideousness of my face. The feeling is utterly delightful. I then realize what I have lost; it is much of my life. The constant dull ache in the pit of my stomach is replaced by a crescendo of pain that stabs everywhere. Every nerve end is damaged. My anger and grief are indescribable. My bone graft caused intense pain but it was nothing compared with this. Drugs will not give relief this time. A massive void opens up inside me. An image of someone who I will call Amanda enters my mind in an attempt to fill it. I want to talk to her, I want to confide in her; I want to explain. The pain intensifies and I know that there is nothing that I can do to relieve it. My feelings and my emotions, that have been suppressed for so long, escape at last. It is like the breaching of a dam and the pain is intolerable.

I go home, change and get on to my exercise bicycle. The perspiration pours off me but the exercise gives little relief. I go to bed in the early hours but I cannot rest. I toss and turn continuously. I drop into a fitful sleep and I awake, still in the early hours, soaked with perspiration. I cannot eliminate Amanda from my mind.

As the days pass, the pain gets worse. I feel that my head will burst. After leaving work, I get into the car and drive home. I scream and yell at the top of my voice to try to bring some relief. My language is vile. The bridge supports on the motorway look inviting but they are protected by crash barriers. Twice I am near to driving at speed up the embankment and then down into a support. It would relieve the horrendous pain but there is a tiny spot of sanity at the back of my mind and I refrain.

This is the start of intense desperation.

When I am alone in the car, I play the same tapes over and over. I lose interest in Radio Four. Chris Farlowe, James Last and Connie Francis almost deafen me.

Sleep is almost impossible. I am used to seven or eight hours. Now I am fortunate to get three. Invariably, I awake before 3 a.m. every morning. My brain is crystal clear and I ache to recover what I have lost. I get up and try to distract my mind with other activities. I find it difficult to initiate recovery. The pain is so intense. The flow through the breach intensifies.

I take up badminton. My fitness improves and I begin to communicate with the other players and the instructors. It is difficult at first. I feel that I have been in a time warp but gradually, very gradually my communication skills improve.

For hours at a time I walk continuously from one room to the other. I understand how a caged animal feels. I ask the same question repeatedly: 'Why? Why? Why?...'. I am unable to find an answer.

I visit Amanda but it is not an enjoyable occasion. I am unable to explain and I leave feeling utterly crestfallen. The pain intensifies.

After several appointments, my doctor begins to understand my problem. He arranges for me to see a psychologist but, apart from talking, he does not know what it will achieve. I am past caring. I desperately need to talk.

The psychologist tells me that I am not mentally ill nor do I suffer from depression. I have low self-esteem and he prescribes art therapy.

I start to face up to my problems. I discover the psychology section in the library that deals with personal problems. I wonder if there are any support groups.

I buy a personal stereo and I try to dance to the music. I am surprised by my progress. I discover that I have some rhythm. I dance for hours, creating more perspiration. I feel I have achieved something and my self-esteem improves. My feelings of ungainliness and awkwardness begin to fade.

An article in a national newspaper catches my eye. It describes the work of a clinical counsellor attached to an NHS plastic surgery unit. She is the only professional counsellor in Britain concerned with facial disfigurement. I resolve to see her.

I undergo art therapy. I receive fifty minutes each week. I draw, I model, I paint and I act an episode from my past. I do not think that these activities alone achieve a great deal but it is sheer bliss to talk to the therapist. I crave for the fifty minutes as an addict craves for a drug. She is young and intelligent. She suggests that I am going through part of my adolescence. She explains how I can dismantle my barriers. This will increase my vulnerability but I must begin to take risks and be prepared to accept rejection. Gradually, very gradually I begin to improve. My outer defence begins to crumble and to contract. At the end of my course, the central core of my problem remains. My therapist explains that it will take many months to overcome. I find this difficult to accept but she assures me that she has given me a sound basis for facing up to and overcoming my problem.

I come across an article in a national newspaper. There is a photograph of a mother and her daughter. The daughter was born with a hare lip. Her mother explains her initial shock, the problems of feeding her baby, and her embarrassment when meeting the public. She found a surgeon whom she could trust and spent twenty years cajoling him to repair her daughter's face. I compare this to the attitude of my own parents. Anger returns.

My first workshop at Changing Faces. There are eight of us; some are young, female and intelligent. I find that I can talk to them. Their own disfigurement causes them similar torment. There is empathy between us. They feel mutilated, withdrawn and lonely. Their eyes depict the demoralization and the incompleteness of their lives. They feel the same as I do. This gives me enormous relief. I am not unique. There is a male teenager who, initially, is full of bravado. He does not admit to his problems. Later, however, he shies from some of the workshop activities. He is unable to speak in front of a group. I know exactly how he feels.

I make an effort to talk to females and find that I am accepted. My progress is slow but I find that my conversation begins to improve.

I attend dancing classes. The new skills improve my social confidence and also teach me to touch and be touched by others. The latter may seem trivial to many but to be touched by a female without a look of horror on her face is a new and delightful experience. I find that I begin to enjoy social functions.

I find a friend who is willing to listen to me. She offers understanding and advice. I talk to her often. It helps me enormously.

I am given the opportunity to join the committee of a local charity. After several months I am appointed treasurer. This gives me a sense of responsibility. I get on well with the members of the committee and they accept my accounting efforts. I sense a feeling of respect.

I have attempted to explain some of my experiences caused by disfigurement and also some of the actions that have helped me to adjust to being a normal and rational human being. It is a difficult process. Thoughts of my disfigurement have faded but they will never disappear completely.

I have discovered that it is difficult for many, including professionals, to even begin to comprehend the psychological effects caused by a facial malformation. Similarly, as someone who started life with a severe disfigurement but is now living with a face that has been surgically perfected, I find it is almost impossible to describe adequately the magnitude of the gulf that exists between the two extremes. It is simply more than a universe of difference....

Chapter 7

James Harden

James was born in Coventry in 1979, an identical twin. He had hypertelorism of his face from the top lip to the forehead. He has just finished his GCSE exams and plans to work in the wholesale industry.

I was born on 18 April 1979. The hypertelorism of my face went from my top lip to my forehead. My twin, Robert, had an extra little toe on his left foot, which was removed after some pressure from our mother. The orthopaedic surgeons did not want to remove it; their comment was: 'It would be a great "talking point" at school as he got older.'

Our mother was told when she was fourteen weeks pregnant that she was having identical twins. We had a very happy and loving childhood. We have an older brother who was two years old when we were born. We were good babies and slept a lot.

When I was born, the medical staff at the hospital in Coventry had never seen anything like me before, and did not quite know what to do. I spent the first twenty-four hours in the intensive care unit (ITU) as they didn't know if all the tubes inside my nose and throat were all there. The first eight weeks of our lives were spent visiting many surgeons in Coventry, including plastic surgeons and ear nose and throat specialists.

All our friends, and the children we went to play school with just accepted the way I looked. Our GP was very good and found out about a surgeon in Oxford. We saw him when we were three months old. He was wonderful to my parents and said it was important that I looked 'normal' when I went to school. He would see me again when I was one year old.

Off we went again to Oxford and this time we saw a surgeon who specialized in craniofacial deformities. He said straight away what he would do. I was seen, along with Robert my twin, every six months, having numerous tests, X-rays, scans etc., until I was three years old, when the surgeon had a special talk with my parents about the high risk factor of the operation. They were talking about a one in fifty chance of blindness and brain damage and a one in thirty chance of not coming through the operation. My parents decided that they would have to take the risk as they did not want me to suffer traumas caused by other children, and so that I could lead a normal life. The surgeon said I was the first child on whom he had done the operation.

My first operation took place in June 1982; it lasted nine hours. I don't remember being frightened in the hospital. I suppose at that young age you do not really know what is going on and just accept things. It was quite a job. The top of my forehead and skull and the scar cartilage were removed; the two halves of my skull were wired together and my eyes moved to the correct position. They took one of my ribs and formed my new nose. Everything went very well and they were pleased. Mum and Dad said that when they came into the ITU at 6.15 p.m. I looked so much like my twin Robert and they just cried with relief that I was all right.

I could not see for eight days, but, again, apparently I just accepted this and never once said, 'Mummy I cannot see.' When my eyes did open, I said, 'I see you Daddy,' and again there were a lot of tears not only from my parents but also from the medical staff. I think this was the point where Mum said she just gave the surgeon the biggest hug ever!

When I returned home after three weeks, it was lovely weather and I was thrilled that I had 'a nose at last'. I could wear a pair of sun glasses, which had obviously never stayed on before and I used to get upset about it as my brothers didn't have this problem.

I wanted to go back to play school straight away. At first, some of the children would not talk to me. I had no hair and had this huge scar that went over the top from ear to ear, and, of course, a nose. One girl would not come near me. She said, 'that's not James.'

My days in infant school were very good but, when I went to the junior school, there were children who did not know me. I started to receive the bullying that went on for the next five years. Things like being called 'spastic', 'mental' and, worst of all, 'squashed nose,' this really used to hurt me. I had six operations by this time, becoming more frightened each time, and having my nose altered at each operation. So, when I was called this sort of name I was very hurt. The older children would not let me play with them and I became very lonely, and, because of all the time I had missed from school, my studies suffered.

This was the time when I started to be very naughty at home and became withdrawn. When I was ten years old, I went through a very traumatic patch and my behaviour was terrible at home. My parents eventually found out what was happening at school and had to see the head mistress to get it all sorted out. Of course, the niceness only lasted for a few days and then I was bullied again. Mental bullying is far worse than the physical kind.

At this point, the surgeon wanted to leave any more surgery until I was about twelve years old, but, of course, when he heard what was happening, he saw me again straight away. He had always asked me every time I saw him if I was having any trouble with other children. Further surgery was arranged straight away, and he said, 'we'll stop them bullying you.'

By the time I was fifteen I had thirteen operations altogether, each one more painful than the last. My skull has been opened up six times in all and I have had bone grafts from the back of my skull to my cheek bones, eye sockets and nose, because this is the hardest bone and would be stronger in the case of childhood accidents etc.

At my last operation, more rib bone and rib cartilage was used to define the shape of my nose. The cartilage was to give the mobile piece on the tip of the nose.

My days at comprehensive school have been quite good. I have had one particular friend called M since I started play school and he is still my best friend today. He is the only person who has never passed any comment about how I look or called me names.

I have not had any bullying as such at comprehensive school, but I do so want to be noticed and liked and I do silly things sometimes to get attention. I have been rude to teachers when all I was trying to do was attract their attention. When I have been struggling to understand something, I have had comments from teachers like: 'Shut up and go and sit down.' This really hurts me. If only someone would give me some time and not keep pushing me away.

I find learning difficult and perhaps my behaviour is down to frustration because of this. I am really struggling and do not work as hard as I should because I cannot cope.

I play the keyboard and have taken exams and passed with a distinction and merits, so I must have the ability to retain knowledge. Perhaps it is because I get individual attention from my music teacher. She is very patient with me. I don't always get the timing right for the first few times of playing a new piece but I get there eventually. I have the ability to discard the music after a few times of playing because I can remember it. My dad used to really help me a lot when I first started playing, but, over the years, this has waned as I get frustrated because I am not getting something right, and then we start shouting at each other.

I get very hurt inside when Dad and I fall out because I love him terribly but I think he finds it hard to accept my incapabilities.

People still stare at me when we are out and this really upsets me because I just want to look normal. I noticed a few weeks ago that my left eye is lower than the right one and became quite upset about this, but my mum reassured me that it wasn't too bad, although I was still upset. That side of my face is quite different from the other. Mum says that when you look at my face through a mirror this deformity is really obvious. This is how I see myself.

I have just started work on a two-year training scheme, learning about the wholesale business. So far, everyone has just accepted me as I am and no questions have been asked yet but I suppose these will come. I really hope that now my life can start to be more normal. Adults accept people as they are. When I had the interview, the Manager said he wanted me straight away. He took me at 'face value', which to me is important. Now I have to prove that I am capable of learning the business. It's what I want to do, so, hopefully, I am going to surprise everyone and at last I will be treated like everyone else.

I love meeting people and I'm very friendly. I have a part-time job a couple of evenings a week where I meet people from all over the world. I do a bit of entertaining and I really love this part. After all I'm up there on the stage and 'getting attention'. Everyone accepts me as I am.

I know I should be better behaved at home. My dad gets so frustrated with me when I'm having tantrums, which seem to last anything from a couple of days to a couple of weeks. I don't know why I get like this and I cannot seem to stop myself; then I settle down again.

I love my parents and my brothers, but even they are horrible to me at times. My twin is a lot cleverer than me and sometimes I feel that he is liked more because of this. I also feel at times that there is no-one who likes me.

James' mother writes about 'coping with James'

Life has been very stressful coping with James. Having the trauma of all the operations and the high risk factor involved has really torn us apart at times; but, when he comes out of an operation it seems all worthwhile.

I support James a lot, much to the dislike of his brothers and dad. I don't feel sorry for James; I just know how he feels. Whether it is because of a mother's intuition or not I cannot say. I have stayed with him at all times in the hospital, which has upset the other two boys. They have always been very loving towards him during this time and when he comes home.

He is just beginning to realize that he does still have a deformity on the left side of his face, which we have always noticed, and when you look at him through the mirror it is so obvious and, of course, this is how James sees himself. He doesn't have the view that other people have by just looking at him normally.

James' behaviour really is exasperating at times. He has terrible tantrums, but I firmly believe this is out of frustration, and I am sure that now he is growing up and is working he will calm down and become more mature.

I suffer most in the few days before James goes into hospital, as I know that once we get there I have to be strong for him. I do not let the family know what I am going through as this would only upset them even more. My husband is strong at this time, but on the days James has an operation he totally goes to pieces. I have had to ban him from coming to the hospital on the day of the operation as I cannot cope with James and his dad at the same time. He usually comes to visit James at night after he's had a couple of telephone calls from me letting him know James' progress.

James hates needles even after all these years and he really is petrified when they want to take a blood sample. The hospital staff are wonderful with him, especially the theatre staff. At his last operation he screamed in the anaesthetic room and refused to let them inject him until he had seen the surgeon and was convinced that he really was there.

The worst time for me was his first operation, not knowing whether we would still have him at the end of the day, but what really upset me was the fact that they were going to shave all his hair off. I just broke down at this point. It was rather silly as it would grow again, but that really was the final straw.

At times, I am so torn at home when James is having tantrums. These seem to happen every few weeks and last for anything up to two weeks at a time. Because I have to support the other two children as well as my husband at the same time, I really have to be the mediator between the four of them, which is very stressful. There are times when I feel I cannot cope any more with the stress, but at the end of the day everything is fine.

Underneath, James is a very loving and caring person. He does a lot of music work with young children and is well thought of by the other teenagers in his music group. The children love him. He seems to have an ability to understand them. He is also very good with older people.

All in all, I would not have changed my life even if I could.

Part Two

Acquired Disfigurement

Chapter 8

Anthony Oakeshott

Anthony Oakeshott is aged 49 and lives in London, working for a large corporation. He was injured in an accident in his child-hood, which left him with a facial paralysis on one side of his face.

How do I feel at present? Certainly not brimful of confidence in my future. More truthfully, I am resigned to having to live with facial injury for the rest of my life and coping as best I can with the problems that stem from it, resigned to a life that so far has been unfulfilled in many ways.

It's not all gloom of course. I have much to be grateful for when looking around and seeing others' lives. I will try to describe why I feel as I do and my progress so far.

I was a normal seven-year-old. During the summer I was involved in a serious car accident as I was just crossing a road. A friend of mine at this time, Adrian, was also involved. Both of us were rushed to hospital and underwent operations; we both received similar injuries, mine being the worst.

The nursing staff were very kind, attentive and cared for us in every way they could. I was discharged after three months and was left with a partial facial paralysis, much like a Bell's palsy to the right side of my face. Fortunately, there was no apparent facial scarring, just one scar under the right jaw line.

My return to life was not too much of an ordeal. Living in a large apart-ment block, news of the accident soon spread and people expected to see an injury of some sort. I was welcomed home by family and friends and, although I experienced some nervousness, people were supportive and sym-pathetic. One young friend offered me some comics as a gift, which touched me deeply. My experience was shared by my friend Adrian who had also been through this traumatic time, so I did not feel totally alone in this.

There were, of course, some looks of curiosity from other children, which made me feel uncomfortable and confused, not being of an age to be able to handle these situations. Gradually I was accepted, and people around me adjusted to my new appearance. I did, however, encounter some examples of insensitivity from the occasional child who perhaps wasn't as sensitive as they might have been. I recall one boy of my age who made a point of asking at each and every meeting: 'And how is your face Anthony?' Although we didn't meet often, this continued up to the age of fourteen, seven years after the accident! It was a painful reminder at this age of my distinct feeling of being 'different' to others.

My childhood from the age of seven onwards was, overall, a very happy one. Both my parents were very supportive. Of course, both my mother and my father were extremely distraught at my accident and spent many sleepless nights during my hospitalization, but were thankful I was still alive and had come through it, as at one point it was touch and go whether or not I would survive.

I can't quite remember when, but there gradually awoke in me a feeling that I was now 'different' to others, possibly at ten or eleven, I don't know. This feeling would sometimes surface if I was in a mixed group of children. The presence of girls stirred in me latent sexual feelings at the age of ten or eleven and, coupled with this strange feeling of being different, would lead to a distinct feeling of shyness, a feeling carried through teenage years into adult life.

My early school years at primary school had been fairly happy, but, looking back at my later years there, I think my facial injury was beginning to shape my personality. I am by nature outgoing, full of life, and gregarious but remember becoming withdrawn somewhat and reserved and not eager to come forward. My self-conscious feelings were growing, especially as we had little contact with girls because there were segregated classes.

My next school was a Catholic grammar school, which was all boys, so here again there was no contact with girls. At home I had no contact with them either, I lost a sister at a very early age, and, although I had three half-sisters through my father's first marriage, I did not see them often, so I led a rather solitary home life, which probably reinforced my sense of being apart. My father died when I was twelve, so I have not had a strong paternal figure to guide me. The combination of these circumstances could have, to some extent, compounded the problem of feeling inferior from a young age. A healthier home environment for a young lad in my circumstances would have been to be living amongst a large family with brothers and sisters. On a more positive note I was fairly popular as a youngster and had plenty of friends of my own age but all were boys.

Overall, my time at grammar school was a happy one, only marred by a few incidents that were disturbing to me. I remember once being asked to perform a 'pop' song of the day to my class, which went all right. Afterwards, one particularly aggressive boy mimicked my facial expression by twisting his mouth exaggeratedly, which put a damper on things and left me feeling hurt, injured and 'powerless'. I did not know how to retaliate and ignored him. Nevertheless, it reinforced my own feelings of inadequacy.

Another incident I recall was when during a difference of opinion with a class mate, he resorted to calling me 'bosseyed jaw boy', a painful reminder of my injury. Yet again, two boys in class made fun of me by making me laugh at their antics and then laughing directly at me because of my facial paralysis. These incidents were small, and, mercifully, few and far between, but they are still memorable even to this day.

I dated a few girls from the age of sixteen but these friendships were very short-lived. By now I was inhibited by my complete uncertainty about how to handle my self-consciousness at being unable to smile broadly. It's surprising just how important a smile is. I spent most of my time on a date trying to conceal my injury and was reluctant to let go for fear of the girl seeing the extent of the injury and rejecting me. I must have appeared to them as a young man without spontaneity and they soon became tired of my company.

I would bring these problems to my mother time and again. She was always very supportive and would say that the injury was hardly noticeable and that one day I'd meet someone who would accept it.

I remember being on a double date and overheard one of the girls saying, 'He doesn't smile much does he?' Needless to say, this was the first and last time I saw this particular girl.

I left school at sixteen with some formal educational qualifications not knowing what lay ahead and having no clear idea of a career. There was a chance of my entering a journalistic career through the influence of my father who had been a top Fleet Street journalist before he died. Unfortunately, perhaps, I didn't feel I could cope with such a high-profile career as this and rejected it. Whether this feeling of inferiority and lack of confidence was a result of my injury I'm not sure, but, looking back, I feel that it probably played a part, a large part, in my decision.

With an injury like mine at a young age, one doesn't have the strength or the wherewithal to cope with such a problem and I remember seeing myself not in an active role but in a passive one, one where I wouldn't be on show too much. I simply couldn't see myself in the hurly burly of Fleet Street, rubbing shoulders with achievers. I had to find a haven, if you like, a 'safe' position without the pressures of what to a young mind appeared like being in the spotlight.

Stage work, acting and dance were ironically always my first love. This interest probably comes from my mother's involvement in acting and singing and also my grandmother who was a singer. I would dearly have liked to join a ballet school or attend drama classes but this wretched injury, in my mind, put paid to all those desires. My confidence levels in teenage years were not high and for me to participate in one of these activities would have been like climbing Everest. My self-esteem was pretty low and I regarded those youngsters that did participate as somehow being 'normal' and full of confidence compared with my worthlessness. I just simply felt overawed at the thought of having to mix in with a young crowd at drama school and the thought of being on stage for all the world to see my disability was an impossible dream. The best I could do in the circumstances was to join my local theatre club to study the history of theatre and to act as a general helper. This was all right for the short time it lasted, but my inward frustration at not being able to do what I wanted became too much to bear and I left. My mother, bless her heart, suggested I see the Director to see if my injury might be an obstacle to taking part in drama classes but I never found the courage to make the approach.

These frustrations would be manifested in my behaviour at home and my poor mother would bear the grunt (yes, I wrote 'grunt' but mean 'brunt') of my outpourings. These would be nasty scenes with me going on at her about my misfortune and inability to change the situation. She was always very patient and understanding and offered kind words and would encourage me, despite my injury, to give it a go, but I never did. The odds, it seemed to me, were too heavily stacked against me.

My mood swings from even temperament to anger at the damage to my development brought about by my facial injury continued through to my mid-twenties. I sought help from a psychiatrist at the age of eighteen. Although very kind and understanding, he sent me away with a pat on the back, reassuring me that there was nothing wrong with me and to get on with my life.

At sixteen, I went to work for a music publisher and quite enjoyed my time there. The work was pretty mundane, though, and I left after one year. From then to age twenty-four, I had around eight different jobs from photographer, gardener and civil servant, to engineer's assistant in the construction of the Victoria Line. It was a search for fulfilment I suppose. I didn't encounter too much prejudice in all this, perhaps because my work was pretty low grade.

There was an opportunity to become a photographer rather than a backroom boy. This would have meant my attending lavish dinners and banquets, taking pictures of guests. My employer could see I was shy and suggested I might try, but my reserve got the better of me and I declined. I remember feeling much regret and envy at seeing a friend in this company take up the offer and go on to become an active member of the photographic staff. It appears that my facial injury has had a very negative influence on my working potential and my potential as a human being.

I have experienced some insensitivity from others at various places of work. I remember a rather ignorant man joining a conversation I was having with a colleague and then pointedly remarking that it looked as though I had bad toothache. At eighteen, this did not do my ego much good. I overheard a conversation recently in which a member of staff referred to me as 'the one with the funny mouth'. In response, I condemned her for being so insensitive and she apologized.

In my mid-twenties my private life picked up and I met and married a girl. Unfortunately, this did not last long and we were divorced within four years. At this time I secured a clerical post to raise money for a mortgage. I remain in this job to this day. The injury was never an issue in our marriage; however, we were very unsuited. I'm sure that, if I had not been involved in this car accident, my development as a person would have been smoother, leading to a sounder personality with greater understanding and experience of women, and perhaps my choice of partner would have been better. In my situation, girl friends are hard to come by and it was the fear of loneliness that drove me to marry the wrong partner.

At thirty-two, I met a musician. She was disabled and there was instant empathy. We lived together for eight years before parting. She was considerably older than me but my life with her was rich and she taught me to forget myself and think of others. It was perhaps because we had so much in our mutual love of music, theatre and cinema that we got on so well. Here was a person who also had problems. I could at last compete on even terms. This was a very enriching experience, one that I will value always.

I remarried when I was forty-two, but, sadly, this came to an end after five years. Again, my accident was never an issue, it was a case of different personalities, different attitudes to life.

Finally, I want to describe the feeling caused through appearing different to others. I decided to go folk dancing alone. Much trepidation is felt, much nervousness, so much so that it can be a good hour before I venture to enter the dance hall. I have to screw up all my courage before asking a girl for a dance. Invariably we will have just the one dance before she makes an excuse and leaves.

The problem seems to be my inability to smile directly at my partner. I'm therefore robbed of spontaneity; this is mirrored by my partner's behaviour. I attempt half-smiling and feel uncomfortable, as she does, and therefore she makes a quick exit. If you can imagine only one-half of your face working, you might have some idea of the problem. It seems to hold in check all my natural behaviour, laughter, humour and confidence, putting others at ease. This is my problem in a nutshell and one that I learn to live with on a day-to-day basis. It appears that only rarely will people look right through it and allow one to be oneself without reacting negatively.

I have the impression that because I am facially injured, when, for example, I'm at a meeting at work, my opinions do not seem to be taken seriously and people can be quite dismissive. Whether this is a result of being different, I'm not sure, but this sort of experience does make one wonder.

I have had the same GP since a child and so we have a good relationship. He has seen me through the trauma of my car accident. He has always been supportive and knew my father well before he died. He treats all the family, so there is continuity and friendship. I have only once or twice voiced my fears for the future when I was in my late teens and he referred me to a psychiatrist. He has quite a brusque manner but is very kind-hearted. He told me I made too much of my injury and to 'get on' with life.

My mother is now in her eighties but very fit and enjoys good health. She still has an active mind, is very outgoing and has plenty of friends. She cannot understand the difficulty I have with women, in finding someone. She is just unable to appreciate the difficulties involved. 'Surely,' she will say, 'something as insignificant as a half smile shouldn't put off women from liking you. You must keep on persevering and forget the injury.' 'Easier said than done,' I say. We are very close, too close perhaps. Not having a family of my own and finding difficulty in forming relationships, I still, at forty-nine years of age, see her as an emotional crutch. However, my dependency on her is slowly becoming less, but she remains my main confidante.

I now share my house with a male friend of thirty-five years standing, a bachelor with whom I get on very well. Because of my difficulties in forming relationships and all the hassle this entails, more often than not I will go out with him. In some ways perhaps it would be better if I experienced more loneliness as this would drive me more to find a partner. The facial injury has never been an issue in our relationship and, whenever I have mentioned it, he dismisses it as being insignificant and saying that it wouldn't discourage girls.

Chapter 9

Kwasi Afari-Mintu

Kwasi was born in Ghana and works in the music business. He was one of the survivors of the King's Cross Underground fire disaster in 1987, which killed 30 people. He told his story to Piers Dungeon of *The Observer* newspaper in November 1992.

For almost a year after the fire, nobody knew that I existed. The BBC found me. 'Where have you been hiding?' they said. I was on nobody's list. I hadn't even been interviewed for the official report. The others had been treated near the scene of the fire at University College Hospital, but I had been placed far away from the public eye, in Queen Mary's Hospital, Roehampton.

When they finally put me on television, I was dubbed the 'man in the mask', a bit of sensationalism that first brought the word 'compensation' to people's lips. I told them that the most important thing was to ensure nothing like the fire ever happened again.

How much is it worth to have been the most badly burned person in the King's Cross fire, and survive? It's the question everybody still asks me, and, if they don't, it's the one they want to ask. Even before I started to get better, I had offers from women to look after me.... It's very sad.

Thinking about this interview has had me piecing back together the nightmare of the fire and looking at where it's left me. In the process I have learned a great deal about myself, and not a little about the inadequacies of the official record of events.

At about 6 p.m. on the evening of 18 November 1987, I was travelling home from the Compact Discount Centre in Golders Green, a music shop where I worked part-time. My route took me down the Northern Line to King's Cross and then northwards along the Victoria Line to Blackhorse Road Station. It was the evening rush hour and, as ever, the trains were running late.

I arrived at King's Cross just before seven to be greeted on the platform by smoke. As I climbed the short escalator towards the Victoria Line platform, the smoke was already strong enough to sting my throat. It was being sucked across the top of the escalator, which I hurried up, and on up to the Victoria Line to my right.

An elderly man said that he'd seen smoke there when he had passed that way at 10 a.m., so I didn't bother to investigate. I assumed staff had got things under control. When we emerged on to the Victoria Line platform I noticed the old man looked tired after talking and keeping pace with me on the stairs, so I found him a seat and carried on down to the far end of the platform (near the Pentonville Road exit) where I knew I could get into a carriage that would drop me near the 'up' escalator at Blackhorse Road.

Hardly had I found a corner to rest my feet when several firemen came on to the platform shouting, 'Everybody up the escalator.' There was no panic in their voices and, remembering the old man's words, I didn't think it was an emergency. I did hear one fireman say, 'This place could go up in flames at any time', but there was no sense of fear in the other passengers and my mind dwelt instead on devising an alternative means to get home: maybe board the 58 bus, go through Dalston....

So, the fire had been smouldering for at least nine hours, and, contrary to the official report, the firemen had arrived more than two minutes before it exploded into action. I was surprised that not one of them remained to supervise our evacuation. Perhaps they were looking for other passengers to alert.

We passengers did as we'd been told and walked briskly up the escalator towards the ticket concourse. I remember turning back once or twice as we went, realizing that my decision to wait at the far end of the platform had meant that I was among the last to leave. There were only four people behind me: two teenage girls, an elderly man and a middle-aged woman; ahead of us were some twenty people. I remember the ride as unusually slow. There was still no excitement, no apparent need to run.

Picture it: the escalator wall is on our left, we're travelling up the left-hand escalator, one of three staircases. As it brings me high enough to catch my first glimpse of the ticket floor I understand why everybody coming off immediately takes to the right. There, roughly northeast of my position, across the semicircular concourse, and standing beside one of those black sentry boxes used by the underground staff who are checking tickets, is one lone fireman, looking somewhat bulky in his shiny costume and ordering: 'Everybody this way. Everybody this way.'

My mind is still preoccupied with sorting out the easiest bus route home and it occurs to me to go over and ask the fireman, though I am aware of people already crowding around him.

I am next in line to come off the escalator. My left leg makes it, but, before my right can take a firm foothold, there comes an almighty bang, very close to my ears, followed by a blackout and then a blinding flash and searing heat on the left-hand side of my face. A huge fireball appears where the ceiling meets the wall immediately on my left, races across the concourse ceiling and drops directly on to the fireman. I watch appalled as he sort of struggles with it, grappling with this huge ball of fire, trying to get it away from his face and body as he falls to the floor. He is the first man to die.

The official line is that a lighted match started the fire on the Piccadilly Line escalator (way over to my right), that it caught hold of an accumulation of grease, dust and debris beneath the wooden steps, and set alight gases gathered in the cleaning trench there. Well, maybe it did. Maybe the fire started under the Piccadilly escalator and somehow travelled under the floor of the Victoria Line escalators and up behind the wall on my left. I can't say, but the fireball – the flashover as they called it – erupted nowhere near the Piccadilly Line. I have the scars to prove it.

The wooden sentry structure is now burning fiercely, blocking my get-away, and the people closest to the fireman are also overwhelmed. Their burning bodies form the only source of light in the place; no electricity, no windows down here, just blackness and smoke and that ghastly pool of light.

The fireball is followed by an eerie whistling sound that shocks me into action. I move away from the fire, keeping to the wall on my left, when suddenly the glow is added to by a second fireball – again accompanied by that awful whistling that haunts me still – flying so close to the ceiling that the whole ticket floor is lit up.

The second bang is so strong that I am thrown on my tummy very close to one of the stairwells leading out of the station, but, instead of offering me escape, it highlights the desperateness of my situation: someone has piled a load of wood to block the stairs, to block the way out. I recognize pieces of it as the tables of the newsvendor who stands by the taxi rank in front of the main line station. Some time ago I lived nearby and would buy my paper there. But the wood hasn't fallen into the stairwell, it has been deliberately set up as a barricade and is burning fiercely.

I hear later that all but one of the exits had been blocked in this way to prevent people from coming in. That's why the lone fireman on the con-course had been directing people up to the right, the only way out that remained. But where does that leave us? Only one fireman stayed to tell us which was the open exit and he is dead, and the route he had been indicating is now blocked with burning bodies and materials.

I bury myself in the burning exit, trying desperately to get out. That must have been when the fire took hold of my back. I wasn't aware of any pain, just conscious that something was happening behind me. Cries of 'Help! Oh Help!' register and seem to wrench me out of a daze. On impulse I reach down among the burning wreckage to pull myself up away from the exit. That's when the damage was done to my hands. Once again I feel no pain.

In the glow of the fire on the main concourse I make out people – women, they look middle-aged. They are standing stock still, crying for help. One bit of me says go and help them, but the fire has caught hold of everything now, its circling above us and down below touching everything and I know that if I spend a second longer here I'll be dead. I move away, walking heavily round the perimeter of the concourse, looking for the next exit, and all the time I can hear those women pleading.

I find two exits opposite each other. I must have been moving clockwise around the raised semicircular walkway on the perimeter of the concourse. These exits would be Grays Inn Road and Euston Road South. I find they too are blocked and everything is on fire. Then I notice that the fire behind me has started making wild crackling noises like that of very dry burning bush or forest. It looks like a furnace, very bright red. I resign myself to just hanging on in my corner, and wait to be engulfed by smoke, choked and burned to death or – perhaps? – rescued by those firemen who sent us up the escalator through the gates of hell.

I feel very heavy, my legs are wobbly, and I notice that somehow I have lost my right shoe. I am very, very tired, very desperate and I let it all spill out; there is so much, like a tangle of things in my mind, but my first thought is like a prayer. I am asking God, 'What is my fate?'

Then other things come flooding in. Even if I am to escape, will I be maimed for life? Will I be crippled like my father who had a stroke and struggled along in a wheelchair for twelve years until he finally passed away? It was very slow, an awful way to live and die, and I dread it about as much as being burned to death. So then I pray to God for a quick exit and a smooth one: if this be my turn, so be it, but if you want me to live then get me out of here whole.

Just then, as I finish my farewell, scanning to and fro – left and right of the dark spot where I stand, away from the fire coming up to me – I see a glow of artificial light in the dense smoke, way in the distance.

I begin to move again, groping for support from anything, whether or not it's burning. Something keeps telling me 'move, move, move!', so I try, but my bare right foot is not much help and I seem to have lost any sense of direction. Then I see the strange light again. Keep on moving! Keep on moving boy! So I struggle on, only to come upon yet another furnace apparently blocking some stairs.

I tell myself I must go through this fire to get to the light beyond, the only glimmer of hope. But, even though I see this, even though the fire behind me offers no better escape, I make no move. There comes a time when you just can't take any more. In my stressed state I decided to stay where I am and burn to death.

Then, as I stand there hopelessly, these dreadful pleas of: 'Help! Help! Help me! Oh God help me!' reach me again over the crackling of the fire, and I realize I have but a few seconds to move before I too am engulfed in hell-fire. Blindly, I make my way among the burning materials, down two flights of stairs and into the arms of two St John ambulancemen waiting in the Circle–Metropolitan ticket area.

The drama is over, but I don't know it. People rush over, shouting that my back is on fire, tearing my clothes off; skin comes too. I look back to where I came from and see the fire raging on the stairs. Are we safe? There is smoke, but also electric lights. Are we really safe? There are people crying and wailing here, too. I ask myself, repeatedly, are we sure we are really safe where we are?

An ambulanceman assures me and two of them support me. Did I drop off? I think I must have to come to and see two firemen in front of me, neatly uniformed with gloves and helmets. I mutter to myself, their apparent betrayal of us passengers rages inside. I think they see the expression on my face. One offers a word or two of consolation and retreats, but the other seems to want to prove that he cares. Can't he see I'm not interested? But nothing gets this fireman off, so we plod on until another St John ambulanceman comes over and explains that they've radioed for a train for me.

It arrives full of commuters. I stand there in the open door with only my trousers on, held up by the two ambulancemen, a sea of commuters' faces in front of me. There I stand until Farringdon Road. Oh, please let me lie down! They take me to St Bartholomew's Hospital. Questions. More questions. Are they the press? Doctors? They throw buckets of ice-cold water over me. I am shivering, my teeth chatter with cold. It's too late. I was burned long ago. Leave me alone. Let me lie down. Then they must have taken me to Roehampton. I don't remember anything more.

The next thing I hear is my girlfriend, Regina, crying. My head is blown up like a balloon, my hair is gone. They knew anything might happen when she came to me, so they made her look at me through the window first, and that's when I heard her crying. It is the third day. They didn't tell me. They didn't announce her arrival.

How did we cope? They don't allow mirrors in that ward in the burns unit. It keeps the suicides down. It didn't occur to me that she'd been repelled by what she saw. The odd thing was that for a long time I didn't think of myself as sick. I felt OK inside. I'm a strong person physically, and the most important thing was that I didn't change the way I spoke to Regina, the way I treated her. 'What's that? Regina', I say, 'Why are you crying? I'm not dead yet.'

Somehow I calmed her down that day, and then, as time went on, the doctors and nurses were so good, they had a way of building up your confidence. For months I had the impression that I would be returning home in about two weeks, and managed to convince Regina that all that was needed was time. She stuck by me, and does still. When I couldn't eat, she brought me a meal of my favourite things every night, coming from the East End right across London to Roehampton after work, whatever the weather.

Of course, I knew I was burned on the face. I remember running my hand over my head and realizing my hair was gone, but no-one bothered me with how bad I looked. Then, one day – was it just before Christmas? – I managed to get to the loo on my own. I had started by crawling and thought that if I could move my feet up under my body I might make just one step at a time with the help of supports: the bed, the wall... they encouraged you to make an effort, a wheelchair was out of the question.

I made it, and was washing my hands when I just happened to look into the mirror and saw this strange person looking back. I couldn't believe it. I stood there for a while, just rooted to the spot. I just couldn't believe it. In fact, I ran my hand over my face to make sure that I was the person I was looking at, and then I felt very, very sorry for myself. I realized I'd been changed into something else. I hung on to the sink for twenty or thirty minutes and just cried. It was the first time I really cried. I didn't care if anybody came down and saw me. I sobbed.

The lowest point – you may find this hard to believe, it was a small thing but a huge coming to terms with the truth – came later. I'd been doing well, so I thought, well enough to begin really to believe them when they said I'd be home in two weeks, but one thing hadn't changed. I'd always used a straw to drink my tea. It had never occurred to me to use the cup properly, and now, for the first time since the fire, I put aside the straw and made to lift the cup and put it to my mouth; but I couldn't do it. I couldn't even lift a cup from the top of the table. All of a sudden I realized how useless these hands were, and then came the realization of just how far I had to go.

It was Easter before my social worker started making noises about my going home. 'I'm going to get you kicked out of here. You're getting too pampered.' The occupational therapist put me through the hoops. She made me prepare cups of tea for people, cook for myself, and when they realized some things were still too difficult she provided me with aids – a slicing board where I could cut an onion without holding it, things like that. She taught me everything, even how to tie my laces, but I never was able to do that. If I wanted my trainers off, I had to leave them off.

The social worker got me a bedsit and, with a new mask for my face, I left the burns unit for the first time in more than four months. The mask was plastic. I had to wear it to get my face back into shape, to develop the shape to look more subtle. There were a lot of veins coming out all over the place, and they had to be blended into the skin. I still have a few like that on my forehead.

I spent the first day out with a friend buying a few things for the flat and hauling them up with my poor hands to the second floor where I now lived. The next day, a Thursday, I had to come back to Queen Mary's to see the physio.

I gave no thought to the bus trip until I came to get my ticket. My hands being still swollen and bandaged, I couldn't get the money out of my pocket, so I turned to a lady next to me and asked her to dig into my pocket and get me some loose change. It was very embarrassing. The lady paid my fare, showed her travelcard and was gone, not realizing that there was yet another problem to tackle, retrieving my change from the driver's scoop.

Well, I thought about just leaving it, but I needed my change, so I summoned enough courage to ask the driver to deliver the coins into my palm. He gave me a 'What kind of freak are you, you cheeky bastard' sort of look, but I had my way.

The next morning I had an appointment with the occupational therapist and, since there'd be no physical jerks and to show her how well I was managing, I decided to discard my trainers in favour of a pair of smart black walking shoes, accepting the challenge of tying their laces. I got more and more frustrated at my stupid attempts until finally, worried that I'd make myself late, I left them hanging loose, banged the flat door shut and hurried down the stairs.

The next thing I knew, I had tripped and was struggling for dear life with the banisters. Unable to get a grip on them, I fell, rolling down helplessly until I got to a landing. There, managing to sit up I started to cry, but then I stopped. I began to curse the stairs and then burst out laughing, wildly, unfortunately forgetting that I wasn't alone in the house.

I'd met my neighbour, an old lady, the day before. She had volunteered to do my shopping but I'd turned her down, determined to help myself. I guess she'd decided I didn't like her or had heard my laughing and thought I'd gone crazy, for she opened her door, met my gaze and slammed it shut.

At the hospital, the occupational therapist could see I had problems – there was blood on the dressing on my left hand, my laces were undone and blood had clotted on my white socks – I must have cut a very poor figure. Suddenly, it all became too much. I had never cried in front of a lady before and wasn't about to begin now, so I left for the bathroom and stood there looking into the mirror. On my return I tried to smile but wasn't surprised when she hinted that I may have to come back to the ward.

When I first went back to my flat, the first thing I did was to arrange for a friend to come and see me on the Saturday. Then I read deep into the night.

On the Friday I woke up in a better mood and began to look forward to my first weekend at home. Thinking I could do with some money I went down to the bank. On my way I popped into the housing association office. I pressed the buzzer for attention. A lady appeared and when she came over and met me face to face she went straight back out, never to return. I decided to leave too. On going out I surprised two oldies who ran for their dear lives down the corridor.

I was becoming aware of the fear that my masked appearance could conjure. I found a side street and tried to get the mask off. No good; it stuck to me. To encourage me to wear it all the time, the technician had modelled it so that I needed help to get it off. I had to make a decision; either go to the hospital or back to the flat. So much for the freedom I'd so looked forward to.

It was two weeks before they finally took me back in. I was due for surgery anyway, so I wouldn't have been allowed out for a while even if I'd wanted to. I was no longer in the intensive care unit. There was more freedom and I became more cheerful. I could walk down to reception and hang around cracking a joke or two with the nurses.

There'd also be times when something would click in my mind and I'd stay in bed feeling sorry for myself, wanting to be at home but worrying that I'd never be able to cope. Then the occupational therapist would stress that I must be more independent. 'Smile, cry, do whatever you want, but do something positive.' She showed me how to keep my eyes always set on new heights of achievement. That was the only way to get the fire out of my system, to be always on the go.

About a year after the fire, a flat was found for me nearer the hospital and I spent increasingly long spells at my new home between bouts of surgery. Following the advice, I began to go to the gym to get my body into shape and enrolled on a month's course learning how to make music using a computer system. Later I took lessons on the piano now that my hands – locked claw-like at the knuckles – were no good for playing my guitar.

Before the fire I was a record producer. I had come to England from my home in Ghana to step up my business making music for the West African market. I produced tapes which sold through my family's record shops in Kumasi. Here in England I would be able to use more sophisticated equipment....

Things were going well. I made good money. In Africa we have many tribes with many different cultural traditions, very fine distinctions. You have to be part of these musical traditions at their roots to make it work. I've always been a singer. I played in a student group in Africa as far back as 1965. Then a year after leaving school I got into the music business. What I learned from going from place to place – ideas about rhythms that West African musicians from remote areas have been tapping forever – I began translating into something for the more modern African audience.

Since the fire, the people whose music I was producing and selling in Africa have gone elsewhere. The channels are no longer open to me, and I have to get other jobs to pay the bills, which means I have less and less time to make music.

In hospital, I decided to make records that would have a wider audience for West African music, to produce records that put the original ethnic musical message across to a European audience. Many people have tried to do that, and few have succeeded. This lays me open to failure on a personal scale that I didn't know before. It's more risky. I'm more vulnerable.

My new aims are all part of the new way of life that's been forced on me by the fire. Just to live, I have had to become ambitious. Every stage in my journey to recovery is small and there have been many: eating, talking to people, socializing. It is as if I have to create a whole new person.

Life was easier before. I was more carefree. That's why Regina liked me. The old Kwasi did things without really thinking about tomorrow. Now I can't do that. Failure wasn't part of my vocabulary before, now I am continually dissatisfied because the fire has made me less able to achieve the aims I have set myself in my music.

Also, I have become very suspicious of people, partly because people have been suspicious of me. I don't think I'm being oversensitive, I mean, what makes an adult say – so that I can hear – 'Wow, that man, God, he's really ugly'? What makes a person need to say that? If a schoolchild passes me along the road and starts laughing at me, I don't mind. They're not grown-up enough to know what hurt is, but, if somebody on the bus or train stares at me for a long time, or I overhear them say something, it does disturb me.

The old Kwasi is there, somewhere, at the core, but it is not possible for me to get back to him. Sometimes, when my friends come round – friends who I had before the fire – I forget the scars on my hands and I don't see my face. Then I can dwell in my old self for a while. Once I was a very, very confident person. Life was good because it felt good. I had a very high degree of contentment. It was a special thing and a source of envy among some of the guys with whom I grew up. I was lucky, I could channel these energies through my music. The confidence came through doing something I really like.

Now I am sad; my new personality has made me sad. You can say to me that sadness is part of everyone's life, that some of the best black music has been sad music, but I say to you that this African music is happy music. South Africans may use ballads and voices to propagate feelings about apartheid. Americans may use blues to sing about slavery, but in West Africa we're not used to being sad. If somebody passes away, even the funeral is a celebration. So you see what this fire has done? It's taken something of my Africanness away. How would you compensate that?

Chapter 10

Jane Richardson

Jane (not her real name) lives in London. She has suffered from acne from the age of twelve.

I had a number of conflicting feelings when I was asked to write this short piece. On the one hand I felt terror, and a reluctance to go back and examine closely a deeply painful period. On the other, I felt it would be good for me, and would force me to come to terms with an important part of my life. I was right about the pain.

I'm thirty now, and outwardly my life is successful. I'm a lawyer with a good job. I live in a nice part of London in my own flat. I have an active social life with several close friends and many acquaintances. I don't have a partner at the moment, but there have been relationships in the past. I still have acne, but it's more or less controlled by medication. My face bears scars from two decades of acne, but if you don't come too close I look quite 'normal'.

Yet more and more I'm coming to realize how much my difficulties in life – and I do seem to find life a good deal more painful than I'd like – are to do with having had hideous acne. It's obvious really, when you think about it. I have never, ever, seen anyone with skin as bad as mine was. Apart from two circles around my eyes, it often seemed that there was not a millimetre that was not clogged, inflamed, peeling, full of pus or blood. For women and girls, especially, how you look is how you feel. It is particularly difficult because 'everyone has spots' (they don't, actually), so it's hard to acknowledge severe acne as anything different from or worse than what other people have. It's also so tied up with questions of hygiene and cleanliness; somehow it's your fault, you're not doing something right.

Nowadays my skin is not so bad. I still feel that anyone describing me would mention 'bad skin' fairly near the top of any list of my attributes, but close friends tell me (and they assure me they're not lying) that I look fine. I know, though, how profoundly my image of myself is based on how I looked then, rather than how I look now. I know how unclean I feel, how undeserving of respect, how different to others. I feel a freak. This realization is all the more surprising because I don't think I ever had these feelings consciously when my skin was at its worst. Perhaps it would have been better if I had felt the pain more. I might have acknowledged it and learnt ways to deal with it, so that its influence on my life would not have been (as I now feel) so destructive.

A bit of history first. Until I was twenty, my parents lived in the Far East, with my sister and I coming to an all-girls boarding school in England when I was twelve. I don't remember when my acne started, but certainly by the time I came to England it was pretty well established. Despite a variety of treatments prescribed by my GP, my skin got steadily worse throughout my time at school. At eighteen, I had a year off before university, which I spent living in Singapore.

One of my main reasons for doing this was so that I could spend a large part of each day sunbathing. I had the idea, fostered by years of twice-weekly visits to a nearby hospital for ultraviolet light treatment, that the sun was good for my acne. It did have the effect of drying up some of the worst spots, but I suspect that the main 'improvement' was the darkening of my background skin colour so that the contrast was less great, and the spots less visible.

In my first term at university, a saleswoman at a cosmetics counter in a department store suggested a London skin hospital, St John's, and I asked my GP for a referral. At the acne clinic there I agreed to take part in clinical trials for a new acne drug. In the next few months my skin got dramatically worse. At my next appointment, the dermatologist, aghast, took me off the trial and prescribed something I had not tried before. At last, results! Over the next twelve months there was a big improvement, and my acne has been under control since then, but I still take handfuls of drugs every day, and, compared with 'normal' people I think I have very bad skin.

Those aren't the real problems, though. The cruellest legacy of my acne is the profound conviction that I'm different to others, that I am unworthy, that I can never hope for ordinary human happiness. This is not hyperbole. Although I'm using rather dramatic language, I don't think I'm exaggerating. More and more I've come to realize how much I drag my past into my present. No matter what the objective reality, in my heart I think of myself as I was in my teens. I will always be a freak, someone deeply unworthy, someone lurking on the fringes of humanity, always an observer, never a participant in life. I've come to acknowledge my deep-seated assumption that anyone meeting me for the first time must be filled with repugnance and pity. In conversation, they are fighting not to be revolted or distracted by the way I look.

These realizations are all the more surprising to me now because, in fact, I don't think I experienced my adolescence (for which read 'my acne') as a particular trauma. I remember the endless pills, the washing, the bathing, the scrubbing, the nightly applying of creams, the constant changing of pillowcases and towels, the inspecting, the squeezing, the peeling of scabs, the relentless sunbathing, the UV lamps, the hospitals . . . but I don't remember what any of it felt like. I was a robot going through the motions. The most accurate way to describe it is as a complete blank, a nonevent. I don't remember feelings, I don't even remember much pain; it's as if I don't remember being alive. Instead of having an adolescence, I just had a void. I do have specific acne-related memories, of course, but somehow those are memories of things, not feelings.

I think now that I had this strange numbness because I'd have been overwhelmed if I had experienced my real feelings. They would have been too unbearable, so I denied them and buried them. Now, in adult life, often in the most unexpected way, occasional agony reminds me of the monster lurking below. 'Our Jane looks bonny', commented my grandmother a few years ago at some family occasion, after she hadn't seen me for some months; I fled from the table in tears. 'You look so pretty', a man told me last week; I felt deeply sad. I know these weren't appropriate reactions, but compliments are the most forceful reminder of my permanent unconscious pain about the way I look.

I've been trying to dredge up memories to give an idea of what it was like for me as an adolescent. It was astonishingly hard to find anything. The girls and teachers at my school were kind; I wasn't bullied, and my skin was never an issue, but there were occasional, small things: my best friend, when I was eleven, 'Your nose is just like a strawberry, and it's even got the black bits'; or, later, my five-year-old brother refusing to kiss me because I was 'too spotsy'; children asking, 'Mummy, has that lady got chickenpox?'; some misdemeanour on my part, and my father's contemptuous rage, 'Look at you standing there with your spots hanging out.'

I remember going to buy my first eyeshadow, imagining the cashier thinking scornfully: 'Good heavens, can you seriously believe this is going to make the slightest bit of difference?' I remember, when I was about seventeen, my mother standing before me weeping; words were unnecessary. I was calm, reassuring: 'It's all right Mummy, don't cry, it doesn't matter.' I remember the consultants at St John's trailing after me in the corridors, summoning their colleagues for a look: 'It's very rare that we have a case as bad as yours to treat.' Then, after I'd finally started to respond to treatment: 'Your face last time was just one big pustule, wasn't it?'

I find it heartbreaking now to think how I unquestioningly accepted my lot. 'Jane is very mature for her age', said my school reports. I should have been screaming, raging, fighting. Instead, there were intricate routines I devised for me to deal with it on a practical level. I daydreamed a lot: I had lots of fantasies of skin peeling; someone would discover something to remove the top half-inch layer of my body, and I would step out, fresh and smooth-looking like girls in magazines; or someone would invent a way of removing the flawless skin of corpses – teenage victims of road accidents perhaps – and substitute it for mine.

Boys were out of the question, of course. At the time I don't think this was particularly noticeable, either to me or to anyone else. There weren't exactly a lot of opportunities at a rural all-girls boarding school, and most of my friends didn't have boyfriends either. Of course, in my mind, it was different; I was different. My fantasies weren't about me and the few boys I knew, but of a fictitious smooth-skinned me and improbably handsome men; the better-looking the man, the more my own beauty would be affirmed. I recall only one 'real' fantasy, and it seems to me now almost unbearably poignant. 'You're so beautiful', said my imaginary lover, stroking and kissing, not my face and lips but my neck, the only place he might have found a few inches of unblemished skin.

Now, as an adult, I sometimes think I'm obsessed with my appearance: I'm ugly; I'm hideous; people are staring. Thoughts of my unattractiveness have intruded upon and ruined intimate moments with men; and, of course, add countless complications to the whole issue of romance and sex. Part of me knows that my obsession with the way I look is narcissistic and self-indulgent, an excuse for not getting on with my life. There's no reason at all for me to dramatize things like this. I look fine now, and of course I have a right to hope for things that other women have, but it's incredibly hard to rewrite my image of myself, to turn away from the past and look into the future. I would dearly love my appearance not to be a constant painful issue. I'm working on it, but it looks as if it's going to be a very long haul.

Younger sister's account

I don't really know what to say about Jane's acne; it was always just there. I do remember little incidents, though, like the time our family went away somewhere on a day trip on the train. For some reason, it was a 'special' day, probably because we hadn't seen our parents or our brother John for some time. John was cute then (he was about five) and very cuddlesome, but that day he refused to touch or kiss Jane because 'she's all spotsy'. I remember seeing Jane's face going all red, and seeing her chin shake and her biting her lip and trying to hold back the tears. If Jane ever did cry, my mother would tut and look cross, and my father wouldn't know what to do with himself, but, really, I didn't really think about Jane's acne and how it affected her. I think I may have even been a little glad when she first started getting really spotty, because that meant I would get more of John's attention; and, anyway, Jane had always been the beautiful child and I was the ugly one.

The awfulness of it all really struck me when I was about seventeen (so Jane was eighteen), and Jane and I were out shopping. People were staring at Jane, in disgust, the way people stare at someone who's deformed. I was furious, and just couldn't believe or understand it and I was seething with anger, but then I remember looking at Jane and seeing that she hadn't noticed the staring, but also that she really was very spotty. I almost cried then, but instead just glared at everyone that looked at her and then rushed home. I didn't say anything to Jane because I hoped she hadn't noticed, and I didn't want her to know and then get upset.

Overall, Jane just seemed to cope with the situation. There were only a few times when I saw her cry about the spots, and I don't think she had anyone else to talk to or cry with about it. I wish so much that I'd been thoughtful enough to give her some support then because it must all have been so terrible, but I think we all just let her cope with her feelings on her own. She had lots of help with the practical or physical side of things; the doctors, the trips abroad to the sun, the extra bath allowance at school and the endless nagging about not eating chocolate, but I for one never let her know that I cared about how she was feeling, because I'm not sure I did at the time, or tried to find out a way to help. I'm so sorry, Jane!

Chapter 11

Lisa Woolley

> Lisa is in her early twenties and works as a nanny in the south of England. She had a very difficult birth, which left her with a facial palsy on one side of her face.

I have a face that does not work properly. This has caused me great hardship in many ways since the day it happened. One of the worse things I have had to cope with is that nobody has ever been able to tell me why I am visibly different. However I am expected to live with it, and this I have done for twenty years out of twenty-five.

I can't really remember the first years of being different. Is this because I have a bad memory or have I just blocked it out? From what I am told I was not a very happy child, quite moody at times. Often I ask myself: would I have been like that if my face had been normal? I will never know the answer.

When I did realize that something about my face was wrong and different, I began to always look down to avoid others looking at me. I didn't really like being with people either, not even my family. Consequently, I became very introverted and lonely, just at the time when I think I should have been developing my own personality.

My operations started from the age of eleven (right at the beginning of secondary school). This could not have been worse timing as I soon discovered that children are the most horrible creatures alive when another child has something wrong with them. I hated school, every minute of it. I was called 'crooked face', 'ugly' and constantly told 'nice legs, shame about the face'. They did not let me forget how I looked.

Adults, too, could be very hurtful. I remember one instance when I was having the dreaded school photo taken. As you can imagine being photographed was not one of my favourite things. The lady took my photo and before I was out of earshot she said, 'Does she always look like that?' This did not do much for my confidence in adults!

I have come to the conclusion that school was the biggest contributing factor to the way I feel about my face now. I left school with only a handful of friends. To be honest, I wouldn't give the others the time of day now because of what they put me through.

College was a better experience because there were only girls in my class and we were not in the main building. This meant I did not have to meet lots of people. My lack of experience in social skills meant that I still feared people. I dreaded situations like walking into crowded rooms because I felt that everyone was staring at me even if they weren't. By now I had had numerous operations on my face all of which were successful but had left me with scars. I still looked very different.

The operations got easier as I got older. I never worried about the actual operations, only what I would look like afterwards. I trusted my surgeon one hundred per cent. If I had not, I would not have had any of them done. My facial condition was not life-threatening but it was socially unaccept-able. The operations were therefore a choice I had to take.

I still have difficulty in accepting my face; one day I hope that I will. However, to be totally honest, I know I will never like it. If I could have one wish, other than, obviously, that this had not happened to me, it would be that the help around today for people visibly different had been available to me when I needed it. I have found that attending both one-to-one sessions and the workshops that Changing Faces puts on to be really helpful. I have started to feel 'OK' about myself in a new way.

Lisa's mother writes

Lisa (I was told later) had a traumatic birth. She was born with the cord around her neck and took a few minutes to yell. We do not know to this day whether this started her face to drop or not. She was also born with a sleepy eye on the other side to the one with which she has problems.

Lisa was not a happy baby. Even at the beginning she did not want to be cuddled or held tight; she did not sleep well. We were living in London at the time, she kept having bronchitis and had eczema. We left London to live in Sussex when Lisa was three years old. Her bronchitis and coughs soon went, but she was left with her eczema and dry skin. I cannot really remember when Lisa's face started to drop. I think it was in the top infants' class. She started to wear her hair long and over her face. We just put this down to adolescence. She was having difficulties with her school work and we found out that she had some form of dyslexia.

We took Lisa to the doctor's. The attitude was 'mother fussing again' but we persevered and she was sent to a neurologist. She had a brain scan, which was normal, so they decided that it was something local between the top and bottom of her face. She was then sent to a marvellous plastic surgeon. We saw him on and off for many years. I have lost count of how many opera-tions she has had. I found this the hardest when I had to sign for every operation, the thought of my little girl going through all of this on her own. We were not encouraged in those days to be with them as much as parents are now.

Lisa always said the operations did not hurt her; she was always such a brave little soul. It was always very hard for my husband and I to agree to these operations. We so wanted her face to be right but at the same time we were very worried about how the operations would affect her. As the years went on she became a moody teenager, never really wanting to go out. This again worried us; she put this barrier up to all that loved and cared for her.

Lisa is a very caring and loyal girl; her love comes out in the way she cares for others. She enjoys her work as a nanny and best of all she loves to travel. She seems far the happiest when she has her rucksack on her back. She has a very strong character and I believe that what she has gone through has helped to form this.

We as parents were very worried and upset to find out, years later, how much she had been bullied at school and for how long. If only she had told us, we would have been able to help her. We have tried many times to find people who could help her, but we always drew a blank. As she grew older, her barrier seemed to get higher and people could not understand why she was like this, when all they could see was Lisa, a loving, caring person. They were not looking at her face; they were looking at Lisa.

By a boyfriend

Lisa's face was never really an issue during our three-year relationship. I have found her very attractive from the first time I met her, right up to the present day.

I guess the only effect it had at all was regarding the way she felt about herself. Lisa was excellent at putting on a strong independent front, which hid a lot of the pain and hurt that she had suffered through being 'different' during childhood. For her own protection, she had developed an incredible skill at hiding her feelings. This may have served her well during the taunting at school, but unfortunately kept me from helping her through feelings that were no longer appropriate. This caused me some frustration as it would for anyone who wasn't allowed to help someone they really cared for.

Lisa's main problem was when people stared at her in the street. This unnerved her, as she tended to think it was because of her face rather than for positive reasons like her very attractive figure or warm, friendly manner. Her low opinion of herself tended to reject compliments from either myself or friends and to expect even a casual glance from a stranger to stimulate thoughts in their minds of pity or loathing. I also found this annoying as not only were my sincere compliments met with disbelief and scorn but she was constantly being hurt by her own imagination, which again I could do nothing about.

Lisa's face has played its part in creating a strong, independent young lady who has achieved much in her life that perhaps would not have been possible without the lessons she has learnt through coping with it. For my part, her appearance in no way influenced my feelings for her, as indeed it shouldn't in any relationship that is based on the really important things in life.

Lisa has still some work to do with regard to her own feeling about herself (as have most people) and I wish her all possible luck with that. As for her future relationships, it will be a very lucky man that manages to spend his life with Lisa and I wish them both the best.

Chapter 12

Living visibly different: a summary

James Partridge

A question of beliefs: the social and cultural background

Living with a blemished face or body in late twentieth-century western society seems to offer few attractions, if the incessant messages that bombard our brains and psyches from all sides are to be believed. The constant refrain is how important is 'the body beautiful'; with it comes success in all manner of activities. We are told that social status, sexual attractiveness and financial rewards accompany those who cultivate the right shape and complexion. Glittering products and experiences are promoted on the strength of these assumptions, from cosmetics to sun-drenched holidays, from instant coffee to fashion clothes. For those in search of beauty, cosmetic surgery is available at a price, but strive we should; the glamour of Hollywood and the high life is held out as the epitome of heaven on earth. 'You can't be serious.' I am.

Just to make matters worse, visibly different faces and bodies are frequently used to characterize the evil side of human nature. Perhaps it has always been so; the demons of mythology and early history are frightening archetypes. Today's literature and global movies seem to rely on the simplistic link; suspicion, villainy, evil and wrongdoing are portrayed by characters with disfigured faces and even disfigured names. For example, 'Scar' is the baddy in Disney's *The Lion King*. In *Batman Forever*, the latest Hollywood blockbuster for children, the character 'Two-Face' is half-'normal', half-grotesque, to represent a split personality. The half-face, which is scarred, is hideously threatening, signifying the dark side of his psyche, which is hardly an association that will help the acceptance of those who are significantly visibly different.

On the face of it, then, living with an imperfect face or body is bound to make for feelings of inferiority and low self-esteem and would seem likely to result in a second-class life; or is it?

This is the question wrestled with by so many parents of children born with a disfigurement, and so many people who acquire it. This chapter brings together the central themes of this Section and offers pointers for success in the ring; the wrestling analogy is not so inappropriate. The half-Nelson of personal and cultural assumptions is a hold that *can* be slipped out of, *if* you have luck, know-how, fortitude . . . . All the contributors testify to that. My hope is that this chapter and the rest of the book will convey some of the lessons.

The personal statements in this Section demonstrate in potent terms how profound is the struggle that disfigurement can engender, not just for the individual affected but also for family and friends and, surprisingly perhaps, for almost everyone who becomes interested in it. Disfigurement is complicated for all of us because it rocks the cultural boat. It raises questions about whether the cult of appearance is morally acceptable. Is it fair to demean those whose faces are marked or misshapen any more than it is to belittle someone with a different coloured skin or who uses a wheelchair? Most of us would answer 'no' but are powerless (or so we think) to do much about it.

I am daily seeking the power to confront this issue. I find the glamour side hardest to change, but I think we can sensibly aspire to remove the fear factor around disfigurement. To tackle the stigma means spreading knowledge about the causes and effects of disfigurement, most importantly among the younger generation. It involves raising the awareness of employers, government and the media about unusual appearances. We must argue that the simplistic imagery of disfigurement needs to be replaced and sensitive behaviour promoted. It will take time and may not entirely succeed. It has to be done.

In the meantime, while these long-term educational efforts go on, those who are visibly different will continue to wrestle with their own particular set of beliefs about their futures. The acquisition of 'positive beliefs' is crucial. Marc Crank states how important it was for him that his family never let him believe that his disfigurement rendered him a lesser person; in contrast, Lisa Woolley's school experience illustrates how a powerful teenage peer group reduced her self-belief and left her angry in the conviction of her own worthlessness. Other writers mention key reinforcers (Kathy Lacy's nanny, for example) and crucial underminers (the crowd at the end of the road for Maureen Williams). In Jane Richardson's acne experience, her self-image was reduced to deep negativity about herself: 'I'm ugly and there is no hope.'

What are 'positive beliefs'? They are the beliefs that visibly different people need for survival and success in late twentieth-century society. They deny the simplicity of the 'body beautiful' ideology. They value human uniqueness. They assert the value of looking different; it's OK.

Many of the contributors would, I think, agree that they have adopted positive belief statements like this one:

> I have had a unique experience from which I have learned and go on learning. My trials have been and continue to be painful but I am able to rise above them and make my strengths available for sharing with those around me. Some won't want to share, and that's their misfortune. Those who do will be able to mine a rich seam of uniqueness.

Most would add: 'Would that I could have believed this earlier . . .'.

Positive beliefs have to be resilient and must be capable of frequent reinforcement because they are constantly under threat. They have to become firmly embedded in the bedrock of a person's life and this can take many years. Every day a person with a visible difference is exposed to negative messages which are often so subtly conveyed that they get through his or her defences (and sometimes not so subtly: witness name-calling). These undermine the positive; they devalue the supposedly ugly as unattractive and instil 'people like me can't or don't' attitudes.

How can the positive beliefs be engendered? There is no single answer; the engendering happens in many ways but it is usually from outside sources, although occasionally it is from a person's own deep inner convictions. The most common source is from one or more family members, from a parent, partner or sibling. Positive beliefs also come from a friend or group of peers, from a role model or from hero figures. They may come from a professional counsellor or therapist, from a chaplain, priest or inspirational leader. They may be found in a book or a film. For most people, positive beliefs grow from a whole matrix of different forces and relationships.

The resulting inner conviction (and I mean conviction, not just the idea) that disfigurement is not the end of meaningful life doesn't just arrive and stick. Most people find it takes time to convince themselves let alone other people.... Turning points are rarely precise moments in time. Rather they are gradually ('so very gradually' in John Storry's account) reached.

Disfigurement is very likely to be thought about in negative and disempowering terms. A central task for anyone who seeks to help a person who is visibly different is to engender in them these positive beliefs. It is very much a question of empowering them to disassociate themselves from their cultural norms.

Accepting disfigurement: the limits to medicine and surgery

Those who are visibly different can be forgiven for imagining that medicine and surgery will have the answer to their problems. Public expectation about the brilliance of cosmetic surgery is rarely matched by knowledge about the limits of plastic surgery or dermatology. It therefore comes as a shock for most of us to discover that there are limits. If Hollywood stars can have such youthful face-lifts or brilliant nose-jobs, can't I have this scar removed or that deformity corrected? The uncomfortable fact is that I mostly likely can't. Most of the contributors speak of the difficulty they had in coming to accept this.

It may be that discovering this absolute truth doesn't take quite so long today as it used to do; most plastic surgeons and other health professionals have now realized that they must inform/warn their patients at an early stage about their own clinical limitations. Some, however, persist in believing that they have told their patients, when actually they have been heard to say something completely different: 'He said he could make it look a lot better', 'I didn't really know what to ask and so I just don't know what to look forward to' and 'They said there wasn't anything else they could do.'

Even if the clinician does get his/her message across, that doesn't stop most patients (and, perhaps especially, their parents) from dreaming. 'Maybe there is a specialist somewhere in the world who I could get to see (if I can raise enough money perhaps) who will put it right.' This can lead to much searching of soul, clinical literature and bank accounts.

All the personal accounts in this Section bear out the central importance of a visibly different person's relationships with medical, nursing and para-medical staff. Such is the professional status accorded to consultants that it is rare for patients to call theirs 'a great friend' (as Marc Crank does), but equally, today it is less common to find the deferential tones reported in some people's stories, and, hopefully, the warning issued by Alan Chapple that medicine had failed him will not be in need of repetition.

The quality of these professional relationships will crucially determine how quickly a patient (or parent) starts to accept the limits of medicine. The vital truths about their disfigurement will be passed – or not passed – through these contacts. If there is any inconsistency, the patient is liable to notice it: 'but you said last time that you could do....'. James Harden's faith in his surgeon was based on: 'He said straight away what he would do', and he did it. Could Kwasi's low point with his badly damaged hands have been avoided if he had had more information about their prognosis, or did he have to feel that powerlessness?

The art of informing visibly different patients about their situation calls for subtle skills and great sensitivity. It needs to be done in a deliberate fashion, not on an ad hoc basis. More care should therefore be given by professionals to the art of informing.

For example, it is important to avoid the use of misleading language. It does not help to say, 'we'll be able to get it better' when, in the patient's mind, better means a full recovery after 'flu. 'Better' in the context of disfigurement usually means 'an improvement' and it is kinder to say so directly. The problem is that 'telling bad news' does not come very naturally. It may seem preferable to keep the patient in an optimistic frame of mind. Indeed, not to maintain hope is tantamount in some medical minds to admitting defeat and thereby shattering the illusion of omnipotence. In my mind, this is not good clinical practice because the patient may well be deprived of the facts that will start the process of accepting their disfigurement as permanent. They need to be able to discover that medicine is only part, albeit a big part, of the solution to their disfigurement.

The role of the family

Helping patients who are visibly different to come to terms with their situation cannot be done successfully without ensuring that their immediate family is also supported: parents, siblings, partners and children. In all the accounts in this section, the family features prominently and it doesn't always provide the sustaining support that might be ideal. Sometimes, the feeling is that the family members are still searching for a magical solution and thereby slowing down the acceptance process for the visibly different person. Sometimes, family members seem to be oblivious of the emotional pain involved; sometimes they can see and feel it but don't know what to do about it and so are wracked with guilt.

It is obvious that the family circumstances of all patients with visible differences will greatly affect their rehabilitation. This goes for both congenital and acquired disfigurements. There will be different stresses placed upon the family but, if they are not addressed, the patient will grow up in, or return to, a family that, too, is failing to come to terms with the visible difference.

In my experience, far too often, the clinical team gives only cursory attention to the family's needs. The trauma and bereavement of visible difference need to be considered as a family experience. The pain of Jane Richardson's acne or John Storry's deformity was theirs alone to bear; the rejection they felt from their families made the pain that much more severe. Kwasi's recovery called for major professional support because his family circumstances were far from ideal; contrast this with the supportive atmosphere of some of the other accounts.

The positive beliefs that empower people to live creatively with their difference can best be sown and nurtured in the family, but, to do so, family members must genuinely have worked through or be working through their own responses to the disfigurement. Their ability and willingness to recognize that the visible difference may carry with it a stigma, with which they themselves cannot cope, needs to be investigated if possible by health professionals. If there are signs that deformity or scars are viewed with some embarrassment, this needs to be tackled. The family has to be willing to be seen with and be totally respecting the visibly different person, but, of course, this can go too far; parents can become overprotective in their desire to help. It's a question of balance, and the right balance will shift as time passes.

It is also evident that some, perhaps many, families are not sure how best to give support and are anxious that they don't say or do the wrong things. They need to have access to advice and support, and their worries need to be picked up at clinics or on the wards. A major challenge for the future care of visibly different people is to be able to recognize and address the needs of the patient's family. Holistic care needs to embrace not just the whole person but the whole family.

Social relationships and skills

Visible difference complicates all social encounters from the most fleeting to the most intimate. Anyone who has had a spot in a conspicuous place on the face has an idea what it might feel like to carry a permanent, and perhaps stigmatizing, blemish or deformity. People either look or don't look, they ask or don't ask, they find physical contact difficult, but the spot usually goes away.

It is by no means simple to acquire and develop the interpersonal communication skills, and hence the self-confidence, to cope with the many reactions of other people and to make friends as well. Just one or two encounters that go wrong – like Kwasi's bus driver – can massively threaten confidence and render the individual acutely self-conscious or, at the other extreme, aggressive. John Storry recounts his agonies of self-inversion made worse by his perception of the behaviours of those he met or those who interviewed him. Many of the contributors mention their blighted school lives, with teasing and name-calling being the order of the day, yet seemingly 'out of sight, out of mind' as far as teachers are concerned. Public places and parties are also mentioned as sources of social anguish. Anthony Oakeshott's ghastly double date rubbed salt in his wounds and what he describes as 'my problems with women' perhaps stem from moments like these. Kwasi recounts the laughter from schoolchildren as he passes. 'I don't mind', he says, but if adults do something similar, it hurts.

This area of rehabilitation has, to my mind, been given far too little attention by those who seek to help visibly different people and was at the root of my decision to launch Changing Faces in 1992. Since that time, we have developed some simple methods for helping people with visible difference feel more in control of social encounters. Workshops and training videos are used to demonstrate and instil new communication skills. Rather as you might go to a college to learn cooking skills, so people now contact Changing Faces for training in 'disfigurement lifeskills'. This training starts from a sound understanding of what happens in social interactions where a person with a visible difference is present and then, on the basis of these insights, appropriate communications skills are practised to allow typical reactions to be managed effectively and relationships to be instigated and maintained.

From the accounts in this section and from our work at Changing Faces, I offer here a summary model of the common 'social interaction problems' experienced by visibly different people (whatever their age). I call it the 'SCARED syndrome'; it describes the especially common responses that those with visible differences experience in meeting other people (although I am aware that it is by no means a complete list). Some of the responses are behavioural, some emotional. When meeting someone who is visibly different, other people can feel and/or behave SCARED:

FEELING		BEHAVIOUR
sorry, sympathetic	S	staring, speechless
curious, confused	C	clumsy
anxious	A	asking, awkward
repelled	R	recoiling, rude
embarrassed	E	evasive
distressed	D	deferential

For someone who has a disfigurement, learning how to deal successfully with all these responses is one of the greatest challenges. Many visibly different people will quickly acquire the knack of noticing how awkward, for example, someone they meet is, without knowing how to manage that awkwardness; or, again, the sensation of being stared at can seem distinctly unpleasant (especially when it can happen dozens of times a day). If it is interpreted as hostile and malevolent, the visibly different person can quickly become resentful; whereas, if it is understood as a necessary part of other people gathering information about the visible difference, it will not cause such distress.

To take this analysis a stage further, I suggest that frequently not only are those who meet a facially disfigured person (especially for the first time) likely to display SCAREDness symptoms so also is the individual affected.

The visibly different person may feel and/or behave SCARED:

FEELING		BEHAVIOUR
self-conscious	S	shy
conspicuous	C	cowardly
angry, awkward	A	aggressive
rejected	R	retreating
embarrassed	E	evasive
'different'	D	defensive

The word 'scared' therefore sums up how both parties are often feeling: scared of saying or doing anything to make an unnerving situation worse. For the individual with the visible difference, once trapped in scaredness, there may seem no way out. Teasing and rudeness at school are often reported as inevitable and 'you just have to live with them'. Certain social encounters (perhaps, many) can become a nightmare. First meetings are particularly avoided. Anger can build because 'they' – meaning other people – are so insensitive. Why can't the world be more understanding?

At Changing Faces, we have developed an approach in our workshops and one-to-one sessions, which takes our clients on from this analysis of what can happen in social interactions to develop the skills to break out of SCAREDness. First, we encourage them to realize that it will take a very long time to change society but that they can take the initiative for themselves. They are then asked to find out how to utilize their verbal and non-verbal communication equipment to most effect. Usually, they have to make some changes in the way they present themselves; their clothes, hairstyle, speech, posture, body language, gestures, all have to be reviewed and, if necessary, adapted to convey positive, nonscared messages. The value of eye contact and the magic of the smile is especially emphasized. (Changing Faces will be making these ideas much more widely available over the coming years through booklets, videos and in other ways.) With the acquisition of social skills comes the self-confidence that feeds on itself; social situations cease to be frightening experiences. Friendships can be built and intimate relationships risked. Self-talk also changes in the process from 'I can't' to 'I can'. The chains of disfigurement can gradually be thrown off. . . .

Perhaps the biggest challenge for those who are seeking to help a visibly different person is to promote self-confidence. To evaluate the level of a person's pre-existing social skills, and/or those of his/her immediate family, is essential. How to help them to develop the skills for dealing with playground, party or public place is the next step. Changing Faces is looking at spreading its approach very widely indeed.

Conclusion

As fictional Flat Stanley Lambchop discovered, being visibly different *can* be enjoyable. All the contributors to this section hint at least that this is a real possibility, and, for some, a very real experience. The challenge for those who want to help is to find ways to promote positive beliefs, an awareness of the limits of surgery and medicine, a solid family support system and appropriate interpersonal skills. The rest of this book is dedicated to taking up the challenge.

Section Two

Perspectives from Research and Assessment

Edited by Tony Carr

Chapter 13

Introduction to Section Two

Tony Carr

To complement the insights provided by the personal accounts of living with visible differences presented in Section One, Section Two aims to review pertinent psychological research and to examine the issue of visible difference from medical, social, anthropological and clinical perspectives. Our objectives are to further understanding of the psychological and social processes at work in disfigurement and to inform the reader's approach to clinical practice and assessment.

In Chapter 14, Harris provides a surgeon's perspective on issues of classification in disfigurement. Visible differences are described and their causes are identified. Contemporary surgical techniques, together with their strengths and limitations, are described for a range of problems. Rumsey, in Chapter 15, sets our consideration of visible differences in an historical and cultural perspective. She shows how concepts of beauty have changed over the ages, whereas the importance of appearance has remained fairly constant. She discusses the contemporary cultural emphasis upon youth and beauty and the inevitable obstacles this creates for the visibly different.

Robinson, in Chapter 16, discusses recent psychological research on the effects of visible differences – social, emotional and behavioural – and examines the evidence for the role of such factors as visibility, severity, gender and social support in determining these effects. Walters, in Chapter 17, examines the particular problems faced by children and adolescents in coping with visible differences. She discusses the effects of living with visible differences on attachment, siblings and schooling, and on emotional, physical and intellectual development. Moss reviews individual differences in response to disfigurement in Chapter 18. He looks in detail at a wide range of psychological factors that may mediate the ways in which people cope, including social skills, self-efficacy, shame, perceptions of control and attributional processes. He points out that there is a good deal of evidence on coping processes and individual differences in general, but, as yet, little systematic attempt to use this in the field of visible differences.

The section concludes with two chapters that consider the issue of assessment in clinical practice. Carr points out that appropriate assessment is the foundation of good clinical practice, in facilitating the match between treatment and patients' needs. He reviews the strengths and weaknesses of a range of behavioural and psychological approaches to assessment, including the clinical interview, self-monitoring and relevant psychometric scales and questionnaires. A structured interview pro forma is offered to improve the reliability and validity of the clinical interview. A short section on the assessment of children and toddlers (by Walters) is also included. Roberts-Harry provides a concise review of physical approaches to assessment, ranging from rulers and callipers to computed tomography, magnetic resonance imaging and laser scanning. He describes how developing technology offers real promise of accurate physical assessments that will enable new and more refined surgical treatment of visible differences.

Chapter 14

Types, causes and physical treatment of visible differences

David Harris

Introduction: What are visible differences?

There are two distinct opinions on what constitutes a visibly different appearance: that of the person whose appearance is under consideration and that of others who observe it. In most cases, these opinions differ, and, in researching the interrelationship between quality of appearance and psychological functioning, it is of cardinal importance to remember that it is the person's judgement which is most relevant. 'Visible different-ness' may be regarded as a highly individual concept, which is derived both from self-comparison with the 'normal' appearances of others and from others' expressed opinions. The relevance of observers' judgements lies in how they behave towards people who have visibly different appearances.

What is normal appearance?

There are many physical characteristics such as weight, height, haemoglobin concentration, etc. that can be measured and for which 'normal ranges' are defined. Appearance, however, cannot be measured objectively and there is therefore no defined range of what is 'normal appearance'. It is, as we have said, a matter of personal opinion. The process by which individuals establish a concept of normal appearance is influenced by the cultural environments in which they live and their opportunities to see what other people look like in life, in magazines, in films, on television and so on. We can thus define 'normal appearance' as: an individual concept which is derived from the perception of sameness in the appearances of others. 'Abnormal appearance' is an appearance which deviates from the individual's concept of normal appearance.

Self-consciousness of abnormal appearance

If individuals perceive that an aspect of their appearance is abnormal, one of two things may happen. Either their perceived abnormality causes them little or no concern or it does. In the latter event, they become preoccupied with the feature in question, focusing on that feature in others and becoming sensitive about the possibility that others might be criticizing it in themselves. Such a reaction generates the psychological distress of self-consciousness of appearance. To give an example, plenty of people have large noses and have been teased about them at school. Some, whilst being aware that their noses are unusually large, are unconcerned and ignore their noses in day-to-day living. There are others, however, who become increasingly concerned that their self-perceived abnormality may be obvious to others and that, as a result, they may be less acceptable to their social group. They tend to assume that casual remarks about noses in conversation are aimed at them; they are hurt by friendly 'mickey-taking'; they are embarrassed in front of strangers; and they focus on other people's noses as the first thing they look at 'in order to find someone else with a nose as bad as mine'.

We can thus define self-consciousness of appearance as: 'the distress and dysfunction arising from an awareness of one's own abnormality of appearance'.

Gross and aesthetic disfigurements

If we take the subset of the population who have abnormal appearance, we can imagine a dimension on which, at one end, are people whose abnormalities are immediately obvious to others, and, at the other, are people whose self-perceived abnormalities are apparent to only a few. It is helpful to classify this dimension. Abnormalities of appearance which are immediately obvious to others can be labelled as gross disfigurements and abnormalities of appearances which are obvious to the subject but not obvious to most others can be labelled as aesthetic disfigurements (Harris, 1982a). In the UK, it is estimated that nine in every 1000 adults suffer from 'a scar, blemish or deformity which severely affects ability to lead a normal life' (OPCS, 1988) and two in every 1000 children have 'a scar, blemish or deformity which limits daily activities' (OPCS, 1989). These figures are likely to represent the incidence of gross disfigurement. There are no such data for the incidence of aesthetic disfigurement. However, from a survey of general practitioners, it was estimated that the annual demand for cosmetic surgery in the UK (for the treatment of aesthetic disfigurements) is of the order of 150 000 patients (British Association of Aesthetic Plastic Surgeons, unpublished observations).

It is often assumed, erroneously, that the degree of psychological distress and dysfunction is proportional to the degree of disfigurement. In fact, as is discussed further in Chapters 15, 16 and 18, clinical experience and research show that grossly disfigured and aesthetically disfigured people can suffer the same degree of psychological distress and be equally dysfunctional emotionally and behaviourally. More to the point is whether or not the abnormality can be hidden from other people without causing the individual too much distress from not being able to dress in any way they please and do the things normal-appearing people do; and whether or not the abnormality involves a sexually significant feature such as the breasts to generate feelings of gender anxiety and sexual dysfunction.

Aesthetic dimensions of appearance

We are used to describing human appearance in terms of its constituent bodily and facial features. When these combine in a harmonious way, we describe a person's appearance as 'normal' and 'nice-looking'. When there is disharmony, we begin to perceive appearance as 'abnormal' and 'disfigured'. Patients often describe what they perceive to be wrong with their appearances in terms of aesthetics. Consideration of the aesthetic dimensions of appearance is of substantial help in understanding the motivations of patients who ask for aesthetic plastic surgery and it is also helpful in understanding the dimension of gross–aesthetic disfigurement. The following is a suggested list of aesthetic dimensions of appearance, together with some examples of associated abnormalities of appearance:

Aesthetic dimension Examples of abnormalities of appearance
- presence: partial or complete absence of a feature due to congenital malformation, trauma or surgical amputation; hairiness.
- size: abnormalities of height/weight from genetic inheritance, eating habits, hormonal imbalance, etc.
- shape: deformity due to congenital malformation, tumours, skeletal disease, etc.
- symmetry: breasts–developmental; face–facial palsy, congenital undergrowth (hemifacial microsomia), etc.
- proportion: disproportion of a feature such as the nose or the ears with the face; the breasts, hips or thighs with the figure, etc.
- straightness: crooked nose from trauma, crooked spine from scoliosis, etc.
- tidiness: lax abdominal skin after pregnancy, irregular scars, etc.
- firmness: flabby skin residual from pregnancy, weight reduction, etc.
- smoothness: uneven, coarse surface of the skin from scarring, benign and malignant skin tumours, acne, acne scarring, chronic dermatoses (e.g. psoriasis), facial creasing from ageing, etc.
- colour: discolouration from red/pink/grey scars, birthmarks, skin diseases (e.g. white patches of vitiligo), systemic diseases (e.g. jaundice), tattooing, etc.

These aesthetic dimensions have been ranked in such a way that, as one moves down the list, one moves from appearances which tend to be grossly disfiguring, towards those which tend to be aesthetically disfiguring.

Each dimension has a pair of polar descriptions: for example, 'symmetry' is described as 'perfectly symmetrical' at the positive pole of the dimension and 'grossly asymmetrical' at the negative pole. Depending where the appearance of a particular feature falls on each dimension, so it will be judged to be normal when it is at or near the positive pole, through aesthetically disfiguring to grossly disfiguring when it is at the negative pole. The lower the dimension is in the rank order, the closer to the negative pole an appearance must be if it is to be classified as a gross disfigurement. Also, gross disfigurements tend to be more extensive than aesthetic disfigurements; they often involve more than one aesthetic dimension and more than one bodily or facial feature.

To illustrate the practical value of this classification, let us consider the feature of female breasts. For normal, harmonious appearance, the breasts have to be symmetrical, or almost so, and in proportion with the rest of the figure. Let us now imagine the case of a teenage girl who is self-conscious that one breast is larger than the other. Both breasts are normally formed, so the only abnormality is her asymmetry. If the disparity in the size of her breasts is small, her asymmetry will be towards the positive pole of the symmetry dimension. Most observers will judge her breasts as normal and her perceived abnormality is classified at the aesthetic end of the gross–aesthetic dimension. If, on the other hand, the disparity in the size of her breasts is large, her asymmetry will be at the 'grossly asymmetrical' pole of the symmetry dimension. Most observers will judge her appearance as abnormal and her disfigurement would be classified towards the gross end of the gross–aesthetic dimension.

Now imagine a female patient who has had a mastectomy for breast cancer. Her mastectomy not only has a negative effect on the dimension of symmetry but it also has negative effects on the dimensions of presence (amputation of her breast) and of shape (the deformity of her chest) both of which are ranked higher than symmetry. All observers would judge her appearance as abnormal and her abnormality is classified at the gross end of the gross–aesthetic dimension. It will be shifted still further towards the gross end if the surgeon who did her mastectomy left loose, untidy skin (negative effect on the untidiness dimension) and if subsequent radiotherapy caused discolouration of her skin (negative effect on the colour dimension). Surgical reconstruction of her breast can move all these aesthetic dimensions towards their positive poles by reconstruction of a breast dome and the nipple–areola complex both to restore the breast feature and to normalize the shape of the chest, and modification of the size and shape of the other breast to create symmetry. As a result, her abnormality of appearance is shifted from the gross end of the gross–aesthetic dimension towards the aesthetic end. Remember, however, that the gross–aesthetic dimension is independent of levels of self-consciousness between patients and each of these imagined patients could suffer the same degree of psychological distress and dysfunction from self-consciousness of their self-perceived abnormalities of appearance.

The causes of abnormal appearance

Appearance is dynamic. It changes throughout life, from month to month, from one day to the next and from morning to evening. It is influenced by genetic inheritance, disease, medical and surgical interventions, accidental trauma, the physiological processes of growth and development, reproduction, ageing and fat storage, and the intervention of 'tribal' tattooing and scarification. Facial appearance mirrors physical and psychological well-being such as looking ill, tired, worried, miserable and so on.

It is likely that the cause of an abnormality of appearance will influence both the subject's ability to come to terms with it and the attitudes of observers who see it. For example, a patient who has had a mastectomy for breast cancer may be self-conscious of her abnormal appearance but may rationalize that her abnormality is the price she has paid for her life and this helps her to come to terms with it. On the other hand, a patient who is self-conscious of her disproportionately large breasts about which she has been teased and ridiculed, agonizes: Why me? and finds that, however hard she tries, she is unable to rationalize her feelings of profound self-consciousness (Harris, 1982b). The attitudes of others towards these two patients also differ: others are sympathetic and understanding towards the mastectomy patient but not so towards the large breasted patient. A classification of the causes of abnormal appearance is therefore necessary if we are better to understand how disfigured appearance affects psychological well-being.

Abnormalities of appearance caused by congenital malformation

By definition, these occur pre-memory which influences the nature of the psychological distress and dysfunction which is suffered by the congenitally disfigured person who has no knowledge of what life is like without appearing abnormal. The following is an anatomical list of the commoner malformations.

Malformations of the head and neck

Clefts of the lip and palate are the commonest and occur about once in every 800 live births. Cleft lip is thought to be due to premature arrest in the growth of the embryonic mesoderm of the maxillary processes which fail, on one or both sides of the face, to reach the nasofrontal process from which the nose, the premaxilla and the philtrum of the upper lip form. Cleft lip can therefore be either unilateral or bilateral; for reasons which are unknown, when it is unilateral, it is on the left-hand side in 75 per cent of cases. Cleft lip is twice as common in boys as it is in girls. (Drillien *et al.*, 1966).

Other malformations of the head and neck are rare and too numerous to detail here. They can be due to failure of part of the face to develop such as absence of an orbit and complex facial clefts, or to underdevelopment of part of the facial skeleton such as the cheek bones and upper jaw as in the reacher–Collins syndrome or to premature fusion of the suture lines which separate the bones of the skull as in the so-called craniosynostoses of Cruzon and Apert. The ear may be absent, partially developed or deformed.

The eyes and eyelids can be malformed. Cysts and sinuses can occur from entrapped ectodermal remnants mainly around the ears and on the sides of the neck. Skin tags can remain in front of the ears and on the cheeks. Down's syndrome produces its characteristic features of sloping forehead, oriental eyelid folds, underdevelopment of the upper jaw and enlargement of the tongue (see Mustardé and Jackson, 1988, for detailed information).

Malformations of blood vessels (birthmarks)

Cutaneous haemangiomata (strawberry naevi) are due to delayed maturation of blood vessels. They usually appear as bright red patches about two weeks after birth, grow rapidly into raised red/blue/grey masses during the next six months and then gradually subside over a period of years. The main problem is for the parents because haemangiomatas, particularly when they are involuting, look rather like bruising thereby placing the parents at risk of being stigmatized as baby-batterers.

Vascular malformations (capillary port wine stains, venous haemangiomatas) are always present at birth and persist throughout life. They can occur in the skin of any part of the body but are usually on the face, where their distribution reflects the territories of cutaneous nerves. Port wine stains are strikingly obvious but, probably because they do not cause a distortion of normal shape and contour, quite often the afflicted person is less self-conscious than one might expect (witness former President Gorbachev of the USSR). Capillary vascular malformations may also affect the meninges of the brain to cause epileptiform attacks (Sturge–Weber syndrome).

Venous haemangiomatas are relatively rare and their appearance is often mistaken by other people as indicative of 'a bad heart' or 'blackberry stains'. Even in today's educated society, haemangiomatas and vascular malformations remain shrouded in myth and mystique, causing many mothers to agonize over what they might have done wrong during their pregnancies.

Malformations of the genitalia

These are rare in girls (vaginal agenesis) but common in boys (hypospadias occurs once in every 250 live male births; epispadias is rare). In hypospadias, the urethra terminates proximal to the tip of the glans penis, the foreskin is absent ventrally and there is usually some ventral curvature of the penis causing deflection of the urinary stream and distortion with erection. Although the malformation is not normally visible, surveys of adult hypospadiacs have emphasized its cosmetic disability, particularly at school and later in sexual relationships (Bracka, 1989).

Malformations of the limbs

These are about as common as congenital malformations of the head and neck. They can be due to the failure of part of a limb to form either transversely, such as a missing hand, or longitudinally, such as a club hand. Syndactyly, or webbing, which is the most common malformation, is due to failure of two or more fingers (or toes) to separate. Another fairly common malformation is polydactyly, when an extra digit is present, usually on the ulnar side of a hand or beside the little toe. The constriction band syndrome is of interest in that it is thought to be due to strands of amniotic membrane becoming wrapped around fingers to create deep, encircling grooves and, sometimes, amputations.

Malformations of the trunk

These are mostly those which affect the later development of the breasts, such as asymmetry, accessory breasts and agenesis of the breast (Poland's syndrome when there is associated malformation of the upper limb).

Abnormalities of appearance caused by disease

These abnormalities are more likely to be accepted by both subject and observer on the basis that diseases are a normal part of life. Many diseases are characterized by specific changes in appearance which can be diagnostic. We are concerned here with those chronic diseases, disorders and conditions which alter normal appearance sufficiently to make the sufferer look abnormal to others. It is helpful to classify them in terms of the aesthetic dimensions of appearance and examples are included in the Table of aesthetic dimensions on page 81.

Iatrogenic abnormalities of appearance

Depending on the presence or absence of post-treatment complications which can add to the severity of iatrogenic disfigurement (i.e. disfigurement which is caused by a therapeutic intervention, usually surgical), the subject's response may range from extreme anger ('I've been butchered') to calm acceptance on the basis that the disfigurement is a necessary price to pay for improved health. Treatment of disease can leave a legacy of disfigured appearance, either temporarily or permanently. An example of temporary disfigurement is the loss of hair that can follow chemotherapy or head shaving preparatory to neurosurgery (the presence dimension). Permanent disfigurements resulting from surgical interventions can range from aesthetic to gross.

Most operations leave a scar, the quality of which depends on its direction in relation to the lines of skin tension (the best scars lie parallel), the part of the body which is operated on (scars on the face heal best, those on the back heal worst), the quality of wound healing (haematomas and infection lead to poor scars) and patients' innate characteristics of scar formation (scars tend to stretch in patients with overelastic skin and stay thick and red in patients who have a tendency to form keloid scars). A neat and tidy scar which is level with adjacent skin and is without the untidiness of cross-hatched stitch scars is not usually perceived as an abnormality of appearance. Scars are disfiguring when they are depressed due to tethering to underlying tissues, when their edges are stepped, when they have an irregular outline, when they stretch and when they stay thick and red; that is, when they significantly influence the aesthetic dimensions of shape, tidiness, smoothness and colour.

Gross disfigurements from surgical interventions are mostly associated with the ablation of carcinoma. Radical excision of a malignant tumour, unless it is hidden within the abdominal or thoracic cavity, leaves a deformity of shape. Lumpectomy for breast cancer is an obvious example. Malignant melanoma was, until recently, treated routinely by wide excision and reconstruction with skin grafts, leaving a dish-like deformity, usually on the lower limb or trunk. Many cancers of the head and neck are also treated surgically and, despite modern techniques of reconstructive plastic surgery, patients may be left with gross abnormalities of appearance. This is particularly so following treatment of floor of mouth tumours when resection includes part of the mandible and is combined with a block dissection of lymph nodes in the neck, resulting in deformed shape and asymmetry. Radiotherapy can also cause scarring and discolouration of skin.

Gross disfigurement follows amputations of digits, limbs and the breast for malignant or vascular disease.

Abnormal appearances caused by trauma and burns

As with postoperative scars, post-traumatic scars are aesthetically disfiguring when they are depressed, stepped, have an irregular outline, remain thick and red or become stretched (deformity of shape, untidiness, irregularity and discolouration). In addition, the obviousness of post-traumatic scars is greatly increased if they are greyed and blackened by ingrained dirt (an avoidable disfigurement if dirty wounds are thoroughly scrubbed soon after injury).

Post-traumatic disfigurements are worsened when there is deformity of shape at the site of a fracture or chronic swelling of soft tissues distal to the site of injury (chronic ankle oedema is a common legacy of lower limb fractures). The orthopaedic treatment of fractures by open reduction and internal fixation causes additional scarring. A not infrequent legacy of interventional scarring is the distress suffered by patients with tracheostomy scars or scars at the wrist who are often misjudged as attempted suicides.

Since the introduction of the seat belt law, the incidence of severe facial injuries has fallen dramatically. Nevertheless, they still occur after road traffic accidents, assaults by animals and humans, and industrial accidents. Facial scars usually remain obvious and their disfigurement is worsened if there is an associated deformity of facial features, particularly the eyelids and eyebrows.

Burn injuries are common but, fortunately, most are small and superficial leaving, at worst, an area of skin which is discoloured. In patients with extensive full thickness burns, however, the resulting disfigurement is arguably the worst of all. The reason for this is the biological process of wound contracture: the inherent property of scar tissue to draw together the margins of an area of skin loss. As a result, post-burn scar contractures severely deform bodily and facial features. Skin grafts used to resurface areas of skin loss also contract, to leave an irregular puckered surface and their donor sites are discoloured. The appearance of skin differs in different parts of the body in terms of colour and texture. These characteristics tend to be retained when it is transferred as a graft so that, for example, a skin graft harvested from the thigh to resurface a defect on the face continues to look like thigh skin. The difficulty of matching skin in reconstructive surgery for patients with extensive burns is a major limitation to improving the aesthetic qualities of appearance.

Occasionally, following severe fractures of the facial skeleton, a patient's appearance may be so different from his or her 'normal', pre-accident appearance that the person is unable to come to terms with the 'new' appearance, which is that of a stranger. This can have serious effects on the patient's state of mind and psychological well-being.

As with self-consciousness of abnormal appearance in general, degrees of psychological distress generated by self-consciousness of post-traumatic abnormalities are unrelated to degrees of disfigurement. They can be unexpectedly severe in patients who have been the innocent victims of accidents and in those who suffer from post-traumatic stress disorder (see Moss, Chapter 18).

Abnormal appearance caused by physiological changes

Throughout life, appearance changes in response to the physiological processes of growth and development, ageing, childbearing and fat storage. These changes may produce novel appearances, which are perceived by the individual as being abnormal, particularly if they occur during a period such as adolescence when body image is developing.

These abnormalities are aesthetic, for example: disproportionate growth of nose, ears and breasts in relation to other facial and bodily features; untidiness of lax abdominal skin and striae following pregnancy; laxity of skin in the neck and loss of a clean jaw line with ageing; and disproportionate accumulation of fat in the lower abdomen, hips, thighs or buttocks. Generally speaking, a significant concern of patients who are self-conscious of such abnormalities is that they find other people to be without sympathy and understanding for their problems (Harris, 1982b).

Appearance can also be perceived as abnormal if it causes others to misjudge the person's well-being, character or ethnic background. For example, baggy eyelids due to excess periorbital fat, which cushions the eye, makes a person look tired; ptosis (drooping) of eyebrows, deepening frown lines, heavy nasolabial folds (cheek folds) and drooping of the corners of the mouth due to ageing make a person look worried and miserable; large breastedness is associated with promiscuity; and tattoos are associated with criminality.

The physical treatment of abnormal appearance

Here we must consider prosthetics, cosmetic camouflage and surgery.

Prosthetics are used not only to replace amputated limbs and extracted eyes but also to replace breasts after mastectomy and congenitally absent or surgically excised facial features such as the nose, ears and teeth. Whilst it is possible to reconstruct the breast, it is obviously not possible to surgically reconstruct missing limbs, and the limitations of reconstructive surgery on the face are such that rebuilt noses and ears look far from normal. Generally speaking, prosthetics provide a better alternative particularly nowadays, since the introduction of a new technology known as osseointegration. Metal studs are implanted into bone to which the prosthesis is then securely clipped. Modern silicone technology now enables prosthetists to tailor-make ears, noses and parts of the face to look extremely natural. Patients can even be provided with sets of prostheses to match changes in skin colour during different seasons.

Cosmetic camouflage is a service provided charitably in many NHS hospitals around the country by the British Red Cross. The cosmetics that are used are specially made to be waterproof and adherent in order to last. Cosmetic camouflage is particularly useful for helping people with abnormal appearances due to discolouration such as port wine stains and discoloured scars.

Surgical treatment for abnormal appearances is the subject of reconstructive and aesthetic plastic surgery, the aim of which is to normalize patients' perceived abnormalities of appearance and relieve the associated psychological distress and emotional and behavioural dysfunction. As a general rule, the aim is achievable among patients with aesthetic disfigurements for whom surgery is often a dramatic cure but it is often not achievable among patients with gross disfigurements (Caw and Harris, 1992) although 'having as much done as is possible' can be very beneficial in enabling them to come to terms with abnormalities that are residual. There are several reasons why reconstructive plastic surgery is limited in its ability to normalize gross disfigurements.

Firstly, one can only use the patient's own tissues for reconstruction; those of others (except identical twins) are rejected. Thus, scarring at least, and also possibly deformity, is introduced at the donor sites from which tissues used for reconstruction (skin, fat, muscle and bone) are harvested. Tissue transfer is accomplished in one of three ways:

- by free grafting which depends for success on the graft becoming revascularized by tissues at the recipient site;
- by pedicled flap transfer, whereby the graft retains a vascular attachment to the body during its movement from the donor site, to the recipient site which may or may not be adjacent to the defect;
- by joining the blood vessels of the graft to blood vessels near the recipient defect using microsurgery. Through a better understanding of the anatomy of blood vessels supplying skin, plastic surgeons now have a vast array of flaps from which to chose. Many flaps are now available, which provide not only skin but also muscle, nerve and bone for reconstruction. For instance, it is possible to reanimate a paralysed face by transferring a muscle, such as the pectoralis minor from the chest to the face by microvascular anastomosis and then join its nerve supply to a nerve graft which has been carried across the face and joined to branches of the functional facial nerve (e.g. Harrison, 1985).

Space does not permit a discussion of the indications, advantages and disadvantages of these techniques, but it is important to state that each carries a risk of failure.

Secondly, available donor tissues may be insufficient. This is a common limitation in the reconstruction of severe post-burn scars due to the limited availability of unscarred skin.

Thirdly, as already mentioned, skin never looks the same from one part of the body to another, so there is nearly always a residual disfigurement of discolouration. A recent advance designed to overcome this problem is the use of tissue expanded flaps. A balloon-like tissue expander, made from silicone, is positioned beneath skin adjacent to the area to be reconstructed. Over a period of several weeks, it is progressively expanded by repeated injections of saline, thus causing the overlying skin to stretch (rather like a pregnancy). Once sufficient expansion has been achieved, the expander is removed, the scarred area is excised and the stretched skin is used to reconstruct the resulting defect. Reconstruction by tissue expansion has achieved the greatest utility in the treatment of mastectomy defects and defects of the scalp and forehead.

Another field in which major advances have recently been made is the reconstruction of craniofacial defects and deformities. Following the pioneering work of Tessier during the 1970s (Tessier, 1971), and the introduction of microplates with which to secure repositioned sections of skull and facial bones, craniofacial surgery has now become a specialty of its own and is applied to the treatment of congenital malformations, trauma and malignancies of the skull base which previously were untreatable. Indeed, so successful is craniofacial surgery, that it is the one exception to the general rule that gross disfigurements cannot be normalized. It is now possible, to normalize the gross abnormalities of the craniosynostoses (of Crouzon and Apert) and Down's syndrome.

Techniques of aesthetic plastic surgery are designed to modify shape and form where there is not a problem of major tissue deficiency. The aim here is to normalize disproportion (e.g. by augmenting disproportionately small breasts or reducing disproportionately large ones); to normalize asymmetry (e.g. of the breasts); to normalize unevenness of surface contour by dermabrasion, chemical peeling, skin planing and revision of individual scars; to normalize untidiness of loose skin by dermolipectomy of the abdomen, thighs and upper arms or by face-lifts; to normalize deformities of shape by selective removal of subcutaneous fat using the technique of liposculpture; to normalize disharmony of facial features by modifying the nose, chin, cheek bones and protruding ears, and to normalize appearances which are misjudged by others by reduction of eyebags, face and brow lifts, mastopexy to tighten the aged appearance of empty breasts after breast feeding, and removal of tattoos either surgically or by laser therapy.

As with reconstructive surgery for gross disfigurements, aesthetic surgery carries with it risks of complications, which can produce a less than satisfactory result. Proper patient selection is therefore extremely important. Patients have to be well-motivated which means that they have to be sufficiently self-conscious of their perceived abnormalities of appearance to make it worth their while to take the risks of surgical intervention.

References

Bracka, A. (1989). A long-term view of hypospadias. *Br. J. Plast. Surg.*, **42**, 251–255.

Caw, A. T. and Harris, D. L. (1992). Psychological effects of plastic surgery. Paper presented to the Annual Conference of the British Psychological Society, Brighton.

Drillien, C. M., Ingram, T. T. S. and Wilkinson, E. M. (1966). *The Causes and Natural History of Cleft Lip and Palate*. Edinburgh: E. and S. Livingstone.

Harris, D. L. (1982a). Cosmetic surgery – where does it begin? *Br. J. Plast. Surg.*, **35**, 281–286.

Harris, D. L. (1982b). The symptomatology of abnormal appearance: an anecdotal study. *Br. J. Plast. Surg.*, **35**, 312–323.

Harrison, D. H. (1985). The pectoralis minor vascularised muscle graft for the treatment of unilateral facial palsy. *Plast. Reconstr. Surg.*, **75**, 206–213.

Mustardé, J. C. and Jackson, I. T. (1988). *Plastic Surgery in Infancy and Childhood.* Edinburgh: Churchill Livingstone.

Office of Population Censuses and Surveys. (1988). *Report 1: The prevalence of disability among adults.* London: HMSO.

Office of Population Censuses and Surveys. (1989). *Report 3: The prevalence of disability among children.* London: HMSO.

Tessier, P. (1971). The definitive plastic surgical treatment of severe facial deformities of the craniofacial skeleton. *Plast. Reconstr. Surg.*, **48**, 419–422.

Chapter 15

Historical and anthropological perspectives on appearance

Nichola Rumsey (with contributions from Sarah Bishop and William Shaw)

It is possible to find evidence of the importance and complexity of feelings attached to physical appearance, in particular to those considered beautiful, from a rich variety of sources. These include mythology and legends, anecdotes from history and examples from fairy tales as well as evidence from contemporary society.

There are many legends addressing the subject of beauty and those considered beautiful. Although some of the messages are contradictory, the implication of most is that the possession of beauty is all-important. An enduring Greek legend concerns three powerful goddesses, Hera, Pallas Athene and Aphrodite (Lakoff and Scherr, 1984). All three renowned beauties squabbled over who should receive a golden apple inscribed 'For the fairest' and flung into the midst of a wedding celebration by the goddess of discord, Eris. The trio disrupted the wedding by throwing tantrums, then spitefully attempted to bribe the appointed judge. Among the consequences of their efforts to win the prize was a 10-year war. The underlying tenet of the legend is that the possession of beauty is of paramount importance, to the exclusion of virtually anything else.

Whilst there is no compelling evidence for a relationship between personality and facial characteristics, the notion that character can be read from the face has an ancient and distinguished history. Subscribers to this view have included many great writers, including Cicero ('The face is the image of the soul'), Shakespeare ('There's no art to find the mind's construction in the face') and Oscar Wilde ('It is only shallow people who do not judge by appearance'). Folklore linking aspects of appearance to personality has existed throughout history and persists in current society, for example, in relation to red hair and fiery tempers, high foreheads and intelligence. Fairy tales and children's stories have contributed to pre-existing stereotypes about beauty over the years. In *Snow White*, for example, the stepmother's vanity is central to the plot. She checks her appearance in the mirror daily. Her wickedness stems from vanity and from the fear that her beauty will be eclipsed by that of her stepdaughter.

Evidence for the emphasis placed on physical appearance in current society can be found from other anecdotal sources. Models can become superstars overnight on the basis of their looks. Millions of pounds are spent each year on cosmetic products and diet foods, as people struggle to change their appearance. In western society, we use language that reflects negative attitudes towards those who deviate from the perceived norm, reflected for example in the use of words such as 'abnormality', 'disfigurement', 'impairment', 'disability', 'flawed' or 'different'. These words convey a sense that something is 'wrong' about the way a person looks.

Ideals of beauty

Although beauty has been seen as a predominantly positive attribute over the years, ideals of beauty have changed, both in terms of body shape and facial characteristics. Ancient Egyptian 'beauties' were portrayed with some-what rounded bodies, a very pronounced chin and a jutting lower jaw. For the Greeks in Classical times, a prominent forehead, aquiline nose, weaker chin and a 'cupid's bow' of a mouth were favoured. During the Renaissance, the emphasis was on matched and harmonious facial and bodily propor-tions. Rubens, in the seventeenth century, consistently portrayed plump, fairly muscular women. The fashion of corsetry in the late nineteenth century emphasized the ideal of the hourglass figure.

In this century, the widespread use of the photographic camera and, later, movie and video cameras, has caused a heightening of concern about self-images portrayed in still and moving pictures. Media technology has also created new possibilities of shared conceptions of beauty. Yet still, ideals change over relatively short periods of time. In the late 1950s and 1960s, movie stars were famed for their 'shapeliness', yet in the 1960s and 1970s, female models were consistently portrayed as being particularly slim with small breasts and close cropped hair. Men, on the other hand, grew their hair long and wore necklaces and earrings. In current times, images of fitness are favoured. For females, the trend is for very slim models, who, somewhat paradoxically, possess broad shoulders and quite noticeable breasts. In terms of facial features, the current ideal favours a relatively strong chin, a smaller nose and a less prominent forehead than in previous times.

Despite apparent changes in those attributes considered to be desirable, the pressure to conform to current norms has remained constant.

Attitudes towards appearance

A historical perspective on attitudes towards those with visible differences of appearance has been provided by Shaw (1981). He noted that in Classical times the gods were thought to create 'monstrous' infants, either for their amusement or to warn, admonish or threaten mankind. The power of these beliefs presumably contributed to the practice of sacrificing such infants (and often their mothers) in attempts to placate the gods. In Mesopotamia, congenital deformities were thought to herald future events. Ballantyne (1904, cited in Shaw, 1981) described one tablet, thought to date back to 2000 years BC, which listed a series of optimistic and pessimistic forecasts relating to the appearance of newborn children.

In the Middle Ages, fetal abnormalities which were perceived to have some animal resemblance, were thought to be the product of the union of a human and an animal. It is thought that these beliefs might have been reflected in mythological images such as the Centaur and the Minotaur. The practice of executing such human beings has been recorded as late as the seventeenth century. In 1708, Frederick V of Denmark ruled that no individual with a facial deformity might show himself to a pregnant woman. Other historical explanations of the occurrence of deformity have been ascribed to stellar influences, seminal and menstrual causes, or as the result of the sighting of deformed individuals by a pregnant woman. We might be forgiven for thinking that such explanations are purely a thing of the past, but Shaw noted that even in recent times among some African tribes, a deformed man is prohibited from elevation to chieftaincy. In some rural communities in the Indian subcontinent, families of deformed babies are held in low esteem until certain purifying rituals have been performed. Strauss (1985) noted the occurrence of active infanticide and selective malnutrition of children with birth defects in contemporary China and Brazil.

In western society, many misconceptions persist about visible differences in appearance. In a survey of 200 women reported in 1981, Shaw noted that a variety of explanations were offered to explain the occurrence of birth defects. Many respondents offered quasi-medical explanations, however, others attributed the blame to maternal behaviour (for example, a port wine stain being due to excessive consumption of strawberries or red cabbage during pregnancy). Although folklore formed the basis of a relatively small proportion of the responses, unfavourable preconceptions about the personality of individuals with facial deformities were still prevalent. Bull and Rumsey (1988) suggested that, in adults, although feelings of aversion may still be aroused, these are frequently modified by other emotions such as sympathy and curiosity. Children, however, are less inhibited than adults and more commonly voice their curiosity and disapproval in response to unusual physical features. Grealy (1994) has remarked in relation to teasing that 'the cruelty of children is immense, almost startling in its precision' (p. 5).

What are the origins of prejudices that work to the advantage of those considered physically attractive and to the disadvantage of those perceived as unattractive or visibly different? Various theories have been discussed by Shaw (1981) including instinctive rejection, primitive beliefs, and a process of social conditioning and reinforcement. The instinctual theories focus on the idea that modern people retain a legacy of behaviour handed down from a time when natural selection shaped behavioural as well as physical attributes. From this perspective, facial deformity may be considered to be a visible indication of more profound mental or physical disorder; some degree of instinctual aversion is therefore to be expected. Others have suggested (for example Wright, 1960) that fear results when a normal person's unconscious body image is threatened by the appearance of an individual with a deformity. The visual pattern of a normal face is learned early in life, and another component of instinctive rejection may be the confusion and unease experienced when we see anything strange or abnormal.

Processes of social conditioning and reinforcement are thought to occur when there is pressure within groups to conform to socially defined norms, in this case, relating to appearance. Social norms are perpetuated in many ways, for example through popular imagery. The association of distortions of the human form with evil and terror have been ingrained in our culture through writings, films and comic caricatures. Other pervasive influences in current society in relation to social conditioning and reinforcement include the media and the prevailing ethos of health care provision for those with visible differences.

The media provide us with a constant barrage of messages telling us how we should look and how we should behave. A cursory glance at media advertising reveals implicit stereotypes relating to appearance. Take, for example, the connotations of the words used in the advertising of beauty products. Skin problems are described using terminology such as 'unsightly' and 'blemished'. We are encouraged to use products that will 'cure' these problems, leaving skin 'clean', 'pure', 'sexy' and 'healthy'.

The countless faces on the covers of magazines and books, in films and on television, provide information on our cultural conceptions of beauty. Irony exists in the creation and perpetuation of these images, however, as fashion editors, art directors, creative directors, advertising executives, make-up artists, photographers and models all collude to create an illusion that is made to look invitingly common. The implication of the illusion is that women should strive to achieve this level of physical attractiveness in order to be loved and admired, yet only a tiny minority of people are realistically in a position to achieve this. The pressure is increased by regular articles and features on 'beauty'. Readers are encouraged to criticize their bodies and/or facial features. 'Faults' are identified and suggestions made (frequently involving the purchase of expensive products) as to how these faults might be corrected. Adverts in magazines for cosmetic surgery promise a happier future and looks more consistent with those portrayed on the front covers of magazines (S. Bishop, personal communication). Those with visible differences report that others frequently suggest the possibility of seeking plastic surgery. Grealy (1994) noted that other people were 'always telling her about the wonderful things surgeons can do nowadays!' This left her feeling that the implication behind the comments was that life would improve if she looked like somebody else, rather than herself.

Writers have speculated on the influence of media pressure on body image, which is commonly conceived to be a mental model of the self, an elastic concept, which can fluctuate in response to influences from cultural norms and to feedback from family, peers and significant others. Body image can be thought of as consisting of three components: a socially represented ideal body (such as the representations in the media): an internalized ideal body image (a compromise between the social 'ideal' and genetically determined limitations); and an objective body image (how we feel we look currently). If a person's internalized ideal moves further away from the objective image, the individual may experience distress and lowered feelings of self-worth that further serve to exaggerate the gap between the self and the ideal.

However, the media are clearly not the only influence on social norms and social conditioning in relation to physical attractiveness. The aim of treatment provided by health care professionals in response to concerns over appearance is to make us look 'better'. Similarly, poor aesthetics, rather than poor function, typically serve as the main motivator for patients seeking orthodontic, other dentofacial treatments, or plastic surgery. Surgeons and orthodontists find themselves under pressure to mould people's faces, bodies and teeth according to the dictates of fashion. The pervasive philosophy implied both by the seeking and the provision of these interventions seems to reinforce the idea that an 'improved' appearance will be the answer to a person's problems. For many, considerable benefit may result from these interventions, either as the result of a more positive body image, or perhaps from pleasure derived from aesthetic improvement. However, in terms of perpetuating the myths linking increases in beauty with increased happiness, it seems unfortunate that no additional or alternative support is offered to help people come to terms with their current appearance and to tackle specific problems they may be experiencing (for example, in relation to social functioning or low self-esteem).

Writers have recounted problems relating to changes in the reactions of others to an appearance altered by surgical or orthodontic intervention, or indeed to a lack of change in the behaviour of others, when change had been anticipated. Grealy (1994) felt that, while she was growing up, she was always waiting for the next operation to improve the appearance of her face. When the results were disappointing, she would put her life on 'hold' until the next operation, when surely the result would be better. She believed that once her face was 'fixed', her difficulties would disappear. When, finally, a series of procedures did produce some marked changes in her appearance, Grealy found it very difficult to accept her new appearance. She felt like an imposter; the new face was a mask hiding the real person. Similar experiences have been reported by those whose facial appearance and feelings of identity have been altered through elective surgery, or following surgical repair of trauma injury (see Section One).

New technology and developments in surgical and orthopaedic techniques bring new pressures. We are currently less likely than in the past to see the full range of disfigurements in our everyday lives. Consequently, those who do deviate from the 'norm' are more noticeable and also seem less acceptable. New techniques, for example fetal scanning and neonatal surgery to correct deformities such as a cleft lip, may further increase the idea that abnormality is unacceptable. The proliferation of new procedures, widely advertised in magazines, increases the general acceptability of undergoing surgery to improve one's appearance and serves to exacerbate these trends. Wolf (1990), amongst others, has speculated that, eventually, no self-respecting woman (and perhaps to a lesser extent, man) will venture forth without a surgically unaltered face. As each person responds to societal pressure by seeking surgical correction, the pressure on the rest grows progressively more intense. More and more it seems that visible variation is viewed as an illness to be treated medically or surgically.

Cultural, gender, age and class differences

Within a society at any time there are likely to be differences in how beauty and visible differences are experienced and viewed by others. These differences depend on the race, gender, age, class and previous experience of the individual. Each culture has its own definition of beauty and acceptability (Fallon, 1990). Identification with one's cultural group (whether native or adopted) is important in individuals' perceptions of what is ideal, of how they match up to that ideal, and the pressure they feel to conform to (or disassociate themselves from) that ideal. Strauss (1985) has noted that, in Israel, differences between western Jews, oriental Jews and Arabs exist in their explanations of the origins of birth defects, and in their attitudes towards rehabilitation and community participation. Sargent (1982) worked with Bariba women. In outlying districts, babies born with physical abnormalities – 'witch babies' – would normally be left to die. After migration to urban dwellings, such babies were initially protected in hospitals, but, after returning home, they often became targets of fear, suspicion and consequent physical abuse. In many poorer societies, it is not economically possible to 'repair' or treat disfigurements that are not life-threatening; thus the range of faces that are tolerated and seen as acceptable may be wider than our own. However, Strauss (1985) has pointed out that the impact of cultural and social values on responses to birth defects remains largely uninvestigated.

There are clearly some gender differences in relation to the pressures experienced to conform to societal norms of appearance. Women's self-concepts tend to be correlated with their own perceptions of attractiveness, whereas men's self-concepts relate more closely to perceptions of their physical fitness or effectiveness (Lerner *et al.*, 1973). Women are more likely than men to equate self-worth with 'what they think they look like' and 'what they believe other people think they look like'. Men are often more realistic and accurate in seeing themselves as others see them (Fallon and Rozin, 1985). S. Bishop (personal communication) has noted that gender stereotypes have influenced the research questions posed and the types of studies carried out. The prevailing assumption is that women will be more distressed by problems concerning their appearance. As a result, men may find that they have less opportunity to discuss their feelings, that their problems are not taken seriously, or that they have less access to services than their female counterparts.

Gender differences have also been noticed in relation to ageing. Although, in adolescence, both sexes are frequently distressed by the occurrence of acne, Dull and West (1991) talked of implicit beliefs that, in later life, those age-related changes that are considered normal or natural for men, do not apply to women. Dull and West believe that the prevailing stereotype is that when a man gets old, in society's eyes he can be considered sophisticated, debonair and wise, yet there is enormous pressure on women to disguise the signs of old age and to cover up real or imagined defects. There are indications, however, that more men are becoming appearance conscious. There is evidence of a greater willingness amongst men to dye their hair, to exercise in order to increase muscle definition and outward signs of physical fitness, and to join the waiting list for plastic surgery procedures. Some have linked this change to the increased pressure on middle-aged men to prove their worth in the employment stakes, and to stave off competition from younger potential employees.

However, the process of ageing is a source of fear and despair for many, particularly in western society. Prejudices against age-related changes in appearance manifest themselves in various ways. The elderly are under-represented in the media. Older women (for example, Joan Collins, Racquel Welch) are pronounced beautiful because they are 'defying the signs of ageing'. Attention is paid in the media to techniques for 'turning back the wheels of time' using make-up, surgery and dieting (S. Bishop, personal communication). Conferences and seminars are arranged on the topic of correcting 'deformities' of the ageing face. All this adds fuel to the idea that people in their natural state slip further towards the ugly and unacceptable end of the appearance continuum as they get older.

Other writers have drawn attention to the class divisions that are being emphasized by increases in the uptake of cosmetic surgical and orthodontic procedures. Interventions are expensive and are thus seen as an option only for the 'elite'. In addition, many trusts and purchasing authorities are considering ruling out NHS funding for cosmetic procedures. These pressures are felt by some to contribute to the current moves towards a two-tiered health service in the UK, with physical differences serving as a further discriminator between the rich and the poor.

The current obsession with physical appearance in our society would appear to work to the detriment of many. From the point of view of those who feel disadvantaged by their appearance, we should promote the view that a wider, rather than an ever decreasing, range of physical attributes should be considered normal and acceptable. However, in order to do so, we need to understand how current societal norms are transmitted and perpetuated.

Kaiser and Chandler (1988) believe that these processes occur through relatively unconscious codes of culture. Both historically and currently, the significance of representations of beauty and of beliefs relating to appearance has been their impact on the self-perceptions of affected individuals and on the impressions formed of them by others. It is to a discussion of these topics that we now turn.

Appearance and social interaction: the transmission and perpetuation of social norms

In terms of social interaction, the advantages of having a physically attractive appearance are widely acknowledged. Researchers in the 1960s and 1970s amassed a large body of literature that attested in particular to the benefits of possessing an attractive face. A number of these studies indicated that assumptions relating to personality, intelligence and success are initially made on the basis of our appearance (see Bull and Rumsey, 1988 for a review). Attractiveness was reported by several researchers to have a powerful effect on liking. On the whole, we expect physically attractive people to possess desirable personality traits such as being warm, kind and sensitive. Huston (1974) found that attractive females were chosen more frequently as potential dates than those who were rated as having medium or low levels of attractiveness. Even in studies in which other factors were controlled (for example, attitude similarity), a strong effect attributable to physical appearance was still widely reported.

Much of this early research relied on the use of head and shoulder photographs of attractive and unattractive people and thus, clearly lacked ecological validity. Barnes and Rosenthal (1985), in studying impressions formed by the same and by mixed-sex dyads, noted that when actual people were used instead of photographs, the strong effects of physical attractiveness became diluted by other available information. Interpersonal attractiveness clearly consists of more than physical features. Factors such as self-presentation, clothes, outward signs of personality, competence, and similarity of beliefs and values also play a part in attraction. In addition, there are many examples of physically unattractive people who are successful and popular, especially if they adopt a skilled interactive style that is rewarding to others. Nevertheless, although the picture is more complicated than early research implied, subsequent studies have confirmed the powerful effect that physical appearance frequently has in initial meetings with others. This is increasingly important in a society such as ours in which we change jobs, move house and meet new people with increasing regularity. It is only in a minority of encounters that we anticipate getting to know others in any depth.

What is the process that gives physically attractive people this potential advantage in initial encounters? The clearest conceptualization of the relationship between physical appearance and social interaction was provided in a four-stage model developed by Adams in 1977. Although it represents an oversimplification of the processes that occur, it none the less provides a useful heuristic.

In the first stage of his model, Adams discussed the phenomenon of stereotyping. Stereotypes are knowledge structures that guide the way individuals process information. They are necessary to impose order on the enormous wealth of information available to us in our dealings with others. We develop, through our experience of social interaction and through cultural influences such as representations in the media, stereotypes of what people are like. These 'schemata' act as channels or filters of information, guiding the individual to pay attention to information that fits the schema and to ignore things that do not fit. Cues derived from physical appearance play a crucial part in the stereotyping process during initial encounters. There is also evidence that our subjective assumptions based on schemata or stereotypes influence our subsequent behaviour towards other people.

Adams' second stage examines this process of social exchange. On the basis of our differing stereotypes of people, we behave differently towards attractive people than those we find less attractive. Altman (1977) found that people rated as being highly attractive tend to receive more eye contact, more smiles and closer bodily proximity than individuals rated as being unattractive. It is these stereotyped reactions or patterns of behaviour that are frequently thought to underlie teasing and the use of nicknames, a problem frequently experienced by those who feel disadvantaged by their appearance.

The third stage of the model suggests that, through the process of initial encounters and through the use of stereotypes by others, attractive people develop internalized self-concepts unlike those formed by unattractive people; in other words, they feel differently about themselves. Macgregor (1979) illustrated this view with a quotation from Tolstoy's book *Childhood*:

'I am convinced that nothing has so marked an influence on the direction of a man's mind as his appearance, and not his appearance in itself so much as his conviction that it is attractive or unattractive.'

Research has supported the idea that, for many, perceptions of physical appearance and perceived feedback from others are central to the self-concept (for a discussion of this process in children, see Walters, Chapter 17). Grealy (1994) described how, at the age of 14, she was dependent on the reactions of other children.

> It was their approval or disapproval which defined everything, and unfortunately, I believed with every cell in my body that approval wasn't written in to my particular script ... it was the language of paranoia. Every whisper I heard was a whisper about how I looked; every laugh a joke at my expense (pp. 4–5).

Adams' last stage describes a self-fulfilling prophecy. As the result, in part, of being the recipient of positive social behaviour from others and also from feelings of positive self-worth, attractive people behave differently compared with unattractive people in the course of their encounters with others. In addition, in many social situations, people sense others' expectations of them and, in the interests of smooth interaction, act in such a way as to fulfil those expectations. The motivation is even stronger if the person wants to be liked by the other participant. This implicit pressure on people to play out an expected role is very strong; failure to do so may result in strained interaction, which is unpleasant for both parties. The strain can lead to social withdrawal and constriction of interaction (Pruzinsky and Cash, 1990) and a consequent lowering of self-esteem. Even events that may not relate to a person's appearance will still be interpreted in terms of that person's appearance.

Despite its usefulness as a heuristic, Adams' conceptualization implies that the process of social interaction is more uniform and universal than it is. Deaux and Major (1987) have shown that additional factors affecting the likelihood of a self-fulfilling prophecy include the strength of social desirability cues, the strength and certainty of the perceiver's stereotype, the power of the perceiver over the 'target', etc. In addition, although physical appearance is clearly important in initial encounters, other factors increase in importance in the longer term. Riggio and Friedman (1986) found in a study of the nonverbal and verbal cues that determine likeability, confidence and competence, that physical attractiveness, though initially important, was less influential in the longer term than other social skills such as expressive facial behaviour, speech and gestural fluency. Buck (1984) has suggested that people who are facially expressive may 'turn on' the expressive behaviour of others. Their expressiveness encourages others to be open and frank in return. Inexpressiveness or facial passivity, on the other hand, dampens the expressiveness of others.

The potential of other behavioural variables to outweigh cues provided by physical appearance has been focused on by those who have felt disadvantaged by their physical appearance (see Section One) and more recently by researchers (see Chapter 16). In view of the difficulties of changing the attitudes and cultural standards outlined in the early stages of this chapter, this provides an interesting avenue to pursue.

Conclusion

In conclusion, it is possible to find evidence of the importance ascribed to physical appearance from a variety of sources, including mythology, folklore and the works of great writers. In contemporary society, attitudes and prejudices related to outward appearance are manifested in many ways: through the media, through the processes of social exchange, and even through the provision of health care.

It would be wrong to imply that beauty is always an advantage, or that those with visible differences invariably experience problems. Anecdotes abound of the concern voiced by 'beautiful' people that others seek them out only for their looks, rather than for more meaningful, pervasive qualities. If anyone feels that they are judged purely on the basis of superficial attributes, life may seem empty and feelings of worthlessness may ensue. For everyone, no matter what their level of physical attractiveness, individual differences must clearly be considered (see Moss, Chapter 18). Some people cope well with their own level of beauty, ugliness or 'differentness', while others struggle.

Despite the need to consider individual variation, there are general conclusions to be drawn. For the sake of those who are unhappy with their outward appearance, it is clearly desirable to encourage all members of society to foster an awareness of their own beliefs and feelings about physical appearance, both in relation to themselves and to others. We should strive to engender an understanding of the impact of the representations and beliefs prevalent in society, and transmitted by individuals, on the body image and self-perceptions of those who feel disadvantaged by their appearance. In addition, we should be fostering an awareness of the superficiality of many of our initial judgements of others and the greater value associated with more meaningful qualities and attributes in the formation and maintenance of satisfying relationships.

Subsequent chapters address the issues of helping those who are experiencing problems relating to their appearance to come to terms with their own physical attributes, and to develop alternative skills and techniques to compensate for any perceived deficiencies (see Section Three).

References

Adams, G. (1977). Physical attractiveness research: toward a developmental social psychology of beauty. *Hum. Dev.*, **20**, 217–225.

Altman, I. (1977). Privacy regulation; culturally universal or culturally specific. *J. Soc. Issues*, **33**, 66–84.

Ballantyne, J. W. (1904). *Manual of Antenatal Pathology and Hygiene: The Embryo*. Edinburgh: William Green & Sons cited in Shaw, W. (1981) Folklore surrounding facial deformity and the origins of facial prejudice. *B. J. Plast. Surg.*, **34**, 237–246.

Barnes, M. and Rosenthal, R. (1985). Interpersonal effects of experimenter attractiveness, attire and gender. *J. Pers. Social Psychol.*, **48**, 435–446.

Buck, R. (1984). *The Communication of Emotion*. New York: Guildford Press.

Bull, R. and Rumsey, N. (1988). *The Social Psychology of Facial Appearance*. Berlin: Springer-Verlag.

Deaux, K. K. and Major, B. (1987) Putting gender into context: an integrative model of gender-related behaviour. *Psychological Review,* **94**, 369–389.

Dull, D. and West, C. (1991). Accounting for cosmetic surgery: the accomplishment of gender. *Soc. Prob.,* **32**(1), 54–70.

Fallon, A. (1990). Culture in the mirror: sociocultural determinants of body image. In *Body Image: Development, Deviance and Change* (T. Cash and T. Pruzinsky, eds.), pp. 80–109, New York: Guilford Press.

Fallon, A. and Rozin, P. (1985). Sex differences in perceptions of desirable body shape. *J. Abnorm. Psychol.,* **94**, 102–105.

Grealy, L. (1994). *In the Mind's Eye: An Autobiography of a Face.* London: Arrow.

Huston, T. (1974). *Foundations of Interpersonal Attraction.* New York: Academic Press.

Kaiser, S. and Chandler, J. (1988). Audience responses to appearance codes: old age imagery in the media. *Gerontologist,* **28**(5), 26–32.

Lakoff, R. and Scherr, R. (1984). *Face Value: The Politics of Beauty.* Boston, MA: Routledge & Kegan Paul.

Lerner, R., Karabenick, S. and Stuart, J. (1973). Relationships among physical attractiveness, body attitudes and self concept in male and female college students. *J. Psychol.,* **85**, 119–129.

Macgregor, F. (1979). *After Plastic Surgery: Adaptation and Adjustment.* New York: Praeger.

Pruzinsky, T. and Cash, T. (1990). Integrative themes in body image development and change. In *Body Image: Development, Deviance and Change.* (T. Cash and T. Pruzinsky, eds.), pp. 337–350, New York: Guilford Press.

Riggio, R. and Friedman, B. (1986). Impression formation: the role of expressive behaviour. *J. Person. Soc. Psychol.,* **50**, 421–427.

Sargent, C. (1982). The implications of role expectations for birth assistance among Bariba women. *Soc. Sci. Med.,* **16**, 1483.

Shaw, W. (1981). Folklore surrounding facial deformity and the origins of facial prejudice. *B. J. Plast. Surg.,* **34**, 237–246.

Strauss, K. (1985). Culture, rehabilitation and facial birth defects: international case studies. *Cleft Lip Palate J.,* **22**(1), 56–62.

Wolf, N. (1990). *The Beauty Myth. How Images of Beauty are Used Against Women.* London: Chatto & Windus.

Wright, B. (1960). *Physical Disability: A Social Psychological Approach.* New York: Harper & Row.

Chapter 16

Psychological research on visible differences in adults

Emma Robinson

Introduction

In their efforts to go about their daily affairs they are subjected to visual and verbal assaults, and a level of familiarity from strangers... [which include] naked stares, startle reactions, 'double-takes', whispering, remarks, furtive looks, curiosity, personal questions, advice, manifestations of pity or aversion, laughter, ridicule and outright avoidance (Macgregor, 1990).

At first glance, it would seem that there is scarcely a need to research into the psychology of visible differences, since the problems are self-evident: common sense tells us that a disfigurement will bring in its train a host of psychological problems. The greater the deviation from the norms of the day, the more these problems will loom.

As so often happens, common sense is an enemy of truth. Overall, there is no consistent evidence in the disfigurement literature to suggest that disfigured people suffer long-term psychiatric problems. On the other hand, there is evidence of psychological distress and serious concern about social functioning.

Although there is now a considerable amount of literature on this topic, it is patchy. Researchers tend to focus on one disfigurement type and many have used burn patient samples. Fewer have studied the psychosocial effects of congenital disfigurements such as port wine stains, or those caused by dermatological conditions such as acne, eczema, psoriasis or vitiligo. Those examining effects of craniofacial abnormalities (e.g., cleft lip and palate) tend to report fairly young patient samples. With improvements in surgical techniques, more people are surviving with the disfiguring effects of cancer and, as a result, research in this area is now gathering momentum.

The nature and extent of the problem

Two of the most popular research issues have been attempts to identify the nature and prevalence of problems imposed by disfigurement. The conclusions are that most difficulties experienced are very similar, regardless of the type or cause of the disfigurement, although there is a surprising finding that a mild disfigurement can carry a greater psycholological burden than a more severe one.

When one considers the profound social significance of the face (see Rumsey, Chapter 15) and combines this with society's prejudices towards those with unusual appearances, it is not surprising to find that the majority of problems experienced by facially disfigured people stem from their social encounters and the reactions of others. Interactions with strangers are particularly problematic. Facially disfigured people report difficulties in meeting new people (Porter *et al.*, 1990) and in making new friends (Lanigan and Cotterill, 1989), as well as anxieties about developing relationships with the opposite sex (Noar, 1991; Porter *et al.*, 1990; Rubinow *et al.*, 1987). Many feel that they are discriminated against both in work settings and socially (Porter *et al.*, 1986) and report frequent exposure to stares, hurtful comments and intrusive questions about the disfigurement.

Many complain of feelings of social isolation (Gamba *et al.*, 1992; Rubinow *et al.*, 1987), sense that strangers feel uncomfortable with them (Porter *et al.*, 1986), and feel that in general they are avoided and rejected by others. There are good grounds for asserting that these feelings of avoidance are based on reality rather than paranoia, with ample evidence to indicate that many people do their best to avoid contact with the facially disfigured. Members of the general public have been observed to avoid an interaction with a facially disfigured person in the street (Rumsey, 1983; Rumsey and Bull, 1986). Typically, they will do this by increasing their pace, averting their gaze and attempting to ignore the presence of the disfigured person. Such avoidant behaviour is picked up by the facially disfigured person who may well interpret it as a form of rejection.

Avoidance is often transmitted in a nonverbal fashion, which is difficult to suppress and is conveyed almost automatically (Bull and Rumsey, 1988). People tend to stand further away from somebody with a disfigurement and will often choose to stand on the nondisfigured side of the face if possible (Rumsey *et al.*, 1982).

While facially disfigured people are correct in their assertions that they are avoided, there is evidence to indicate that such avoidance is not necessarily due to feelings of repulsion or rejection, as many facially disfigured people assume. Some studies support the idea that avoidance is more likely to be due to the novelty of seeing a facially disfigured person and consequently a feeling of uncertainty about how to behave (Langer *et al.*, 1976) and/or a desire to avoid embarrassment (Rumsey and Bull, 1986).

Whatever the underlying reasons for such negative behaviour, frequent exposure to these reactions can result in a host of psychological problems, including: social anxiety, lowered self-confidence, negative self-image, depression and lowered self-esteem all of which can have a cumulative effect on future interactions. Feelings of self-consciousness can take over (see Harris, Chapter 14) and people can become preoccupied with their disfigurement and the effects this may be having on others. Such preoccupations can escalate out of all proportion; the person begins actively to search for signs that others have noticed the disfigurement or are feeling uncomfortable. Ultimately, a self-fulfilling prophecy can occur where the person anticipates negative reactions in every encounter and thus behaves defensively, or in a shy or aggressive manner, which in itself invites real negativity from others.

Attempts to cope with the reactions of others can be so trying, or the fear of rejection so great, that withdrawal from social situations, often combined with avoidance of occupational, domestic or recreational activities, is frequently chosen as a means of addressing the difficulties experienced (Harris, 1982). For those in whom total withdrawal is not employed as a coping strategy, many nevertheless seem to spend more time with family members and much less time outside this network (Gamba *et al.*, 1992; Macgregor, 1989; Patterson *et al.*, 1993). Unfortunately for some people, problems can extend beyond casual encounters with strangers and may touch on their intimate relationships. Sixteen per cent of the dermatology patients investigated by Hughes *et al.* (1983) reported their condition to affect their married life. Lanigan and Cotterill (1989) found a small proportion of women (9%) who admitted that they would not reveal their birthmarks, even to their husbands.

Fortunately though, not everyone is doomed to such a bleak future. Rumsey (1983) demonstrated that interactions with facially disfigured people can have positive outcomes; a number of studies have found facially disfigured people to be coping quite satisfactorily. Blakeney *et al.* (1988) assessed a sample of young adults, all of whom had sustained severe burn injuries as children (the majority having sustained facial disfigurement). They were well adjusted psychologically and typical of any other group of persons of their age (i.e. of average intelligence, still in school or employed, getting married, having children and so on). Other researchers using similar population samples report parallel findings (e.g. Knudson-Cooper, 1981; Love *et al.*, 1987). Positive adjustment has also been reported for those with port wine stains (Kalick *et al.*, 1981), cancer related disfigurements (West, 1977, cited in Gamba *et al.*, 1992) and craniofacial deformities (Lansdown, 1990).

Such variability in research findings is not surprising in the light of the small, unrepresentative samples that are often reported and the non-standardized measures frequently used. Many researchers fail to report the validity or reliability of the instruments they use. Larger sample sizes are required to enable statistical analysis to take account of the multiple variables possibly affecting outcome. Nevertheless, several researchers have attempted to identify the factors that influence adjustment.

Factors affecting outcome

Severity of the disfigurement

Contrary to what one might expect, the severity of the disfigurement does not appear to be linked to the degree of psychological distress. Although a variety of different methods have been employed to measure severity (e.g. subjective patient ratings, clinicians' ratings, or total burn surface area/ number of days spent in hospital in the case of burn injuries), the majority of studies have found no evidence of a relationship (e.g. Baker, 1992; Love *et al.*, 1987; Malt and Ugland, 1989). In some cases, a relatively mild disfigurement can cause more difficulties than one that is more major. Some researchers have postulated that this is because, unlike responses to major disfigurement, which are fairly predictable and can be anticipated, responses of others to a more minor disfigurement are much more erratic and less easily gauged. Such uncertainty about how other people will behave can serve to reinforce feelings of anxiety and tension (Macgregor, 1990).

Visibility

Although the severity of disfigurement has little value as a predictor of distress, there is some evidence to suggest that its visibility may have slightly more significance, although research findings have been contradictory. Williams and Griffiths (1991) found visibility to be an important predictor of psychological outcome in burn injured patients. Hughes *et al.* (1983) found 70% of the patients in their sample whose dermatological condition affected their face or hands, achieved high scores on the General Health Questionnaire (see Carr, Chapter 19). Porter *et al.* (1986) found psoriasis patients to be less well adjusted than those with vitiligo. They point out that psoriasis is more difficult to conceal (unlike vitiligo, it cannot be concealed cosmetically), which may contribute toward the differences observed.

On the other hand, White (1982) found no correlation between location of burn disfigurement and the incidence or severity of psychological sequelae, and other researchers have found people with visible disfigurements to have made good adjustments (e.g. Knudson-Cooper, 1981).

Gender differences

Several researchers have speculated that gender differences might exist in terms of adjustment outcome; however, few have investigated this per se. It is possible that, in a society such as our own, where a high value is placed on the physical attractiveness of women, that they are more likely to suffer the negative effects of disfigurement (for discussion of gender differences in relation to the ageing process, see Rumsey, Chapter 15).

Men are less likely to use camouflage make-up to disguise their disfigurements (Lanigan and Cotterill, 1989), which may mean that they adopt alternative coping strategies, resulting in better adjustment. Alternatively, men may have just as many concerns about their appearance but suppress them for fear of them being viewed as a sign of weakness. Brown *et al.* (1988) found no differences in the psychosocial adjustment of men and women to burn injury but found the factors that were important in achieving good quality adjustment varied between the two. In order of importance, the variables that contributed to good quality adjustment in men were: less functional disability, less use of avoidance coping, engaging in more recreational activities, greater friend support and more use of problem solving. For women, more use of problem solving was found to be the most important variable, followed by less functional disability, greater family support and, finally, engaging in more recreational activities. Thus, although no differences were observed in quality of adjustment, it may be that the ways in which men and women achieve such adjustment differ. In addition, it is unknown whether engaging in recreational activities is a cause or an effect of better quality adjustment.

Time as a healer

Some researchers have proposed that positive adjustment to disfigurement occurs naturally over time (see Patterson *et al.*, 1993, in relation to burns patients). Although not a process in itself, the passage of time may allow a number of psychological processes, which are supportive of adjustment, to take place. There is evidence to suggest that adjustment does take place naturally over time in some subjects (Love *et al.*, 1987; Malt, 1980). However, there has been little longitudinal research of adequate quality. For example, Tucker (1987) compared a group of predischarge burn patients with a group of burned outpatients and found differences between the two groups, indicating improvement with time in the areas of anxiety, depression and self-esteem. However, no attempt was made to match the two groups, which were acknowledged to differ on a number of variables, thus making any comparisons of limited value. Apart from the fact that the outpatient group was a totally male sample, none showed evidence of psychiatric history, unlike the predischarge group; this is a factor that has been acknowledged to contribute to poor adjustment (Andreasen *et al.*, 1971). In addition, the predischarge group comprised a consecutive series of admissions, yet the outpatient sample was made up of those attending a follow-up clinic and could not be assumed to be randomly selected.

According to Patterson *et al.* (1993), 'for the majority ... a burn represents a temporary, albeit painful disruption from life's routine, one after which they will eventually resume their normal pre-injury functioning'. These authors appear to have overlooked the long-term studies of burned patients that find levels of anxiety and depression, for example, to be quite high one year or more post injury (White, 1982; Williams and Griffiths, 1991) and even to increase over time (Wallace and Lees, 1988).

Further longitudinal research is needed before any conclusions can be reached regarding the healing effect of time, using a range of congenital and acquired disfigurement samples. The absence of long-term studies is one of the main weaknesses in research in this area to date. Follow-up periods of one or two years are not sufficient to allow researchers to make an accurate assessment of long-term adjustment. In addition, participation rates frequently go unreported, which limits the validity of research findings; it may well be that those who do not respond at follow-up may be those not making adequate adjustment. The difficulties of maintaining a large sample over time mean that some researchers have attempted to tackle the issue using cross-sectional studies. However, subjects are rarely matched on variables that may contribute towards adjustment, other than time, thus limiting the validity of any comparisons made.

Psychosocial support

The expressed need

Psychosocial support is often neglected (although it is recognized by many professionals to be an important part of the rehabilitation process). In a survey carried out to establish the type of professional support available in UK burns units, Wallace (1988) found relatively few units had the resources available to provide professional psychological help to patients. Instead, patients tend to be offered the opportunity to attend self-help groups led by staff and/or patients, or to receive counselling from ex-patients or parents. There is a need for professional help that is largely currently unmet and many facially disfigured people have to rely on family and friends.

When asked about the sort of support they would prefer, Wallace (1988) reported patients to be unanimous in expressing a desire for additional information and support. At discharge, 65% said they would welcome some form of regular self-help meeting and 56% continued to express a need for such support six months on. However, the most popular form of help that patients wanted at six months postdischarge was from professionals, with 88% of patients expressing a preference for this sort, and 50% still expressing the need at the two-year mark. Wallace and Lees (1988) suggest that self-referral may be one way of screening those in need of help. Other research suggests, however, that this is a very unreliable method of screening, since patients may severely underestimate their need for psychosocial help, especially if asked upon discharge (Faber et al., 1987).

Evidence of impact

Social support has been acknowledged as having a positive effect on health in general (Cobb, 1976) as well as a buffering effect on stress (Cohen and Wills, 1985). In a study of head and neck cancer survivors, Baker (1992) found that it positively influenced patients' rehabilitation outcome six months post-treatment. In a sample of 82 well-adjusted port wine stain patients (Kalick et al., 1981), all were reported to receive 'extraordinary support from family members'. The maladjusted adults in the sample of burn survivors reported by Browne et al. (1985) perceived less support from friends, family and peers. Families that are supportive have been found positively to influence the psychological adjustment of children (Blakeney et al., 1990) and social support has also been found to be a critical variable in coping with other conditions such as cancer (see Nelles et al., 1991).

The precise mechanism by which this form of help operates is not fully understood. Argyle (1988) suggests that social support may have a direct positive effect on a person's self-esteem and self-confidence. Indeed, in a long-term study of burned patients, Davidson et al. (1981) found that the influence of family, friends and peers was significantly related to self-esteem, as well as to life satisfaction and participation in social and recreational activities. Further research is needed in order to determine what sort of support is the most effective and for whom. Furthermore, measures are needed which include the *quality* of perceived social support, rather than a simple frequency count of the people available. Orr et al. (1989) examined the effect of perceived support from family and friends on body image, self-esteem and depression in burn injured adolescents and young adults, and found perceived support from friends to be the most critical determinant of positive adjustment in this young patient sample. Brown et al. (1988) found that, although women favoured greater involvement with families, friends were more important for men in terms of psychosocial adjustment.

In addition, there is a wide variation in the capability of each patient's social networks to respond (Davidson *et al.*, 1981). Some family members or friends may feel overwhelmed by the emotional needs of the disfigured person and value training and support themselves. What is more, people are not simply passive recipients of help, they play an active role in eliciting it. There are, of course, individual differences in people's ability to do this (for further discussion see Moss, Chapter 18). Finally, future research should attempt to identify whether there are any negative effects of social support (e.g. overprotectiveness or dependency).

Surgery

Facial disfigurement is perceived as being largely a medical problem. Physical solutions (i.e. surgical or medical interventions) are usually the first type of help to be offered; such treatment can radically alter the social experiences of the disfigured person. However, many facially disfigured people will never be able to have their faces reconstructed to achieve normality. Surgery may reduce the disfigurement and improve the appearance but it is unlikely to be able to remove the disfigurement completely; even when improvements are achieved, visible scarring will often remain. Communicating this surgical reality to patients can be an arduous task and many are unable to take this fact on board. This may be due to several factors, for example, informational overload regarding surgical procedures, possible risks/benefits, and the prospect of future surgical interventions. Medical terminology can lead to patient misunderstanding, especially when combined with a genuine uncertainty on the part of the surgical team about what the result will be. High expectations of what surgery may achieve can, however, lead to negative reactions (Macgregor, 1981; Pruzinsky and Edgerton, 1990).

Reconstructive surgery can take many years to complete and, even in those for whom treatment is successful, this offers no guarantee that psychological problems will be resolved. Correlations are not always observed between satisfaction with surgery and psychological improvement. Lovius *et al.* (1990) found that patients who had undergone orthognathic surgery feared negative evaluation from others no less than before surgery, despite reporting improvements in body satisfaction in the area operated upon. Even after substantial improvement in their acne condition, Rubinow *et al.* (1987) found some of their patients to show a continued lack of self-confidence and sensitivity to social rejection. Although social adjustment has been found to improve in the long term following orthognathic surgery (Barbosa *et al.*, 1993), for some people, problems appear to be deep-seated in years of negative experience, and, if left untreated after medical intervention has been completed, psychological problems may persist (Wallace and Lees, 1988).

Social skills training

It is clear that, as with any single approach, surgical/medical interventions have their limitations. We have seen that problems with social situations are very common amongst those with disfigurement. Fear of rejection and low-ered self-confidence can continue long after physical interventions have been completed; the effect that such negative feelings can have on the interaction process have been discussed. Such observations have led researchers to consider the potential of social skills training as a way forward for facially disfigured people. Rumsey *et al.* (1986) suggest that the social reception of facially disfigured people can be improved by their exhibiting strong social skills. Social interaction skills training has recently been made available by the charity, *Changing Faces*, and its effectiveness as a way of reducing psychosocial difficulties amongst facially disfigured people has been under evaluation. Research findings suggest that people can become more socially confident and less anxious with the aid of this type of training (Robinson *et al.*, 1996). Social skills training thus offers another possible approach to the problems experienced by facially disfigured people. Further evaluative research of this nature, testing a variety of interventions, is needed if the psychosocial needs of visibly disfigured people are to be met.

Conclusion

Research has tended to centre around theory rooted in the medical model, where factors such as location or severity of disfigurement are assumed to be all important. We have seen that severity is not a very useful factor in the prediction of psychological outcome. Although visibility may have more predictive power, results are conflicting and there exists a wide range of individual differences in adjustment. More important is the *perception* of severity and the extent to which people allow this to interfere with their lives (which will be guided by factors such as a person's level of social skills, self-esteem, etc.). The extent to which this happens may well be moderated by other factors such as social and family support.

As well as testing new methods of intervention, it is important that we continue to study those factors that enhance or impede the chances of positive adjustment in order to facilitate the identification of those at risk of developing psychosocial problems and to allow us to direct appropriate means of intervention as a *preventative* measure.

References

Andreasen, N., Norris, A. and Hartford, C. (1971). Incidence of long-term psychiatric compli-cations in severely burned adults. *Ann. Surg.*, **174**, 785–793.

Argyle, M. (1988). Social relationships. In *Introduction to Social Psychology* (M. Hewstone, W. Stroebe, J-P. Codol and G. Stephenson, eds.), pp. 222–245, Oxford: Blackwell.

Baker, C. (1992). Factors associated with rehabilitation in head and neck cancer. *Cancer Nurs.*, **15**, 395–400.

Barbosa, A., Marcantonio, E., Barbosa, C., *et al.* (1993). Psychological evaluation of patients scheduled for orthognathic surgery. *J. Nihon. Univ. Sch. Dent.*, **35**, 1–9.

Blakeney, P., Herndon, D., Desai, M., *et al.* (1988). Long-term psychosocial adjustment follow-ing burn injury. *J. Burn Care Rehabil.*, **9**, 661–665.

Blakeney, P., Portman, S. and Rutan, R. (1990). Familial values as factors influencing long-term psychological adjustment of children after severe burn injury. *J. Burn Care Rehabil.*, **11**, 472–475.

Brown, B., Roberts, J., Browne, G., *et al.* (1988). Gender differences in variables associated with psychosocial adjustment to a burn injury. *Res. Nurs. Health.*, **11**, 23–30.

Browne, G., Byrne, C., Brown, B., *et al.* (1985). Psychosocial adjustment of burn survivors. *Burns.*, **12**, 28–35.

Bull, R. and Rumsey, N. (1988). *The Social Psychology of Facial Appearance.* New York: Springer Verlag.

Cobb, S. (1976). Social support as a moderator of life stress. *Psychosom. Med.*, **38**, 300–314.

Cohen, S. and Wills, T. (1985). Stress, social support and the buffering hypothesis. *Psychol. Bull.*, **98**, 310–357.

Davidson, T., Bowden, M., Tholen, D., *et al.* (1981). Social support and post-burn adjustment. *Arch. Phys. Med. Rehabil.*, **62**, 274–278.

Faber, A., Klasen, H., Sauer, E. and Vuister, F. (1987). Psychological and social problems in burn patients after discharge. *Scand. J. Plast. Reconstr. Surg.*, **21**, 307–309.

Harris, D. (1982). The symptomatology of abnormal appearance: an anecdotal survey. *Br. J. Plast. Surg.*, **35**, 312–323.

Hughes, J., Barraclough, B., Hamblin, L. and White, J. (1983). Psychiatric symptoms in dermatology patients. *Bri. J. Psychiatry*, **143**, 51–54.

Kalick, S. M., Goldwyn, R. and Noe, J. (1981). Social issues and body image concerns of port wine stain patients undergoing laser therapy. *Lasers Surg. Med.*, **1**, 205–213.

Knudson-Cooper, M. (1981). Adjustment to visible stigma: the case of the severely burned. *Soc. Sci. Med.*, **15B**, 31–44.

Langer, E., Fiske, S., Taylor, S. and Chanowitz, B. (1976). Stigma, staring and discomfort: a novel-stimulus hypothesis. *J. Exp. Soc. Psychol.*, **12**, 451–463.

Lanigan, S. and Cotterill, J. (1989). Psychological disabilities amongst patients with port wine stains. *Br. J. Dermatol.*, **121**, 209–215.

Lansdown, R. (1990). Psychological problems of patients with cleft lip and palate: Discussion paper. *J. R. Soc. Med.*, **83**, 448–450.

Love, B., Byrne, C., Roberts, J., *et al.* (1987). Adult psychosocial adjustment following childhood injury: the effect of disfigurement. *J. Burn Care Rehabil.*, **8**, 280–285.

Lovius, B., Jones, R., Pospisil, O., *et al.* (1990). The specific psychosocial effects of orthognathic surgery. *J. Craniomaxillofac. Surg.*, **18**, 339–342.

Macgregor, F. (1981). Patient dissatisfaction with results of technically satisfactory surgery. *Aesthetic Plast. Surg.*, **5**, 27–32.

Macgregor, F. (1989). Social, psychological and cultural dimensions of cosmetic and reconstructive plastic surgery. *Aesthetic Plast. Surg.*, **13**, 1–8.

Macgregor, F. (1990). Facial disfigurement: problems and management of social interaction and implications for mental health. *Aesthetic Plast. Surg.*, **14**, 249–257.

Malt, U. (1980). Long-term psychosocial follow-up studies of burned adults: review of the literature. *Burns*, **6**, 190–197.

Malt, U. and Ugland, O. (1989). A long-term psychosocial follow-up study of burned adults. *Acta Psychiatr. Scand. Suppl.*, **355**, 94–102.

Nelles, W., McCaffrey, R., Blanchard, C. and Ruckdeschel, J. (1991). Social supports and breast cancer: a review. *J. Psychosoc. Oncol.*, **9**(2), 21–34.

Noar, J. (1991). Questionnaire survey of attitudes and concerns of patients with cleft lip and palate and their parents. *Cleft Palate Craniofac. J.*, **28**, 279–284.

Orr, D., Reznikoff, M. and Smith, G. (1989). Body image, self-esteem and depression in burn-injured adolescents and young adults. *J. Burn Care Rehabil.*, **10**, 454–461.

Patterson, D., Everett, J., Bombardier, C., *et al.* (1993). Psychological effects of severe burn injuries. *Psychol. Bull.*, **113**, 362–378.

Porter, J., Beuf, A., Lerner, A. and Norlund, J. (1986). Psychosocial effect of vitiligo: a comparison of vitiligo patients with 'normal' control subjects, with psoriasis patients, and with patients with other pigmentary disorders. *J. Am. Acad. Dermatol.*, **15**, 220–224.

Porter, J., Beuf, A., Lerner, A. and Norlund, J. (1990). The effect of vitiligo on sexual relationships. *J. Am. Acad. Dermatol.*, **22**, 221–222.

Pruzinsky, T. and Edgerton, M. (1990). Body-image change in cosmetic plastic surgery. In *Body Images: Development, Deviance and Change* (T. Pruzinsky and T. Cash, eds.), pp. 217–236. New York: Guilford Press.

Robinson, E., Rumsey, N. and Partridge, J. (1996). An evaluation of the impact of social interaction skills training for facially disfigured people. *Br. J. Plast. Surg.*, **49**, 281–289.

Rubinow, D., Peck, G., Squillace, K. and Gnatt, G. (1987). Reduced anxiety and depression in cystic acne patients after successful treatment with oral isotretinoin. *J. Am. Acad. Dermatol.*, **17**, 25–32.

Rumsey, N. (1983). Psychological problems associated with facial disfigurement (Unpublished PhD thesis), North East London Polytechnic.

Rumsey, N. and Bull, R. (1986). The effects of facial disfigurement on social interaction. *Hum. Learning*, **5**, 203–208.

Rumsey, N., Bull, R. and Gahagen, D. (1982). The effect of facial disfigurement on the proxemic behaviour of the general public. *J. Appl. Soc. Psychol.*, **12**, 137–150.

Rumsey, N., Bull. R. and Gahagen, D. (1986). A preliminary study of the effects of social skills training for improving the quality of social interaction for the facially disfigured. *Soc. Behav.*, **1**, 143–145.

Tucker, P. (1987). Psychosocial problems among adult burn victims. *Burns*, **13**, 7–14.

Wallace, L. (1988). Abandoned to a 'social death'? *Nurs. Times*, **84**(10), 34–37.

Wallace, L. and Lees, J. (1988). A psychological follow-up study of adult patients discharged from a British burn unit. *Burns*, **14**, 39–45.

West, D. (1977) Social adaption patterns among cancer patients with facial disfigurement resulting from surgery. *Archives of Physical Medicine and Rehabilitation*, **58**, 473–479. Cited in Gamba, A., Romano, M., Grosso, I., *et al.* (1992). Psychosocial adjustment of patients surgically treated for head and neck cancer. *Head Neck*, **14**, 218–223.

White, A. (1982). Psychiatric study of patients with severe burn injuries. *Br. Med. J.*, **284**, 465–467.

Williams, E. and Griffiths, T. (1991). Psychological consequences of burn injury. *Burns*, **17**, 478–480.

Chapter 17

Problems faced by children and families living with visible differences

Elizabeth Walters

Birth and early days

Advances in antenatal screening mean that the birth of a baby with an undiagnosed physical defect is more unexpected than a decade ago. An intellectual understanding of the statistical risks fails to prepare parents emotionally for such a devastating blow.

Solnit and Stark (1962) first likened the parental experience to mourning, with grief being expressed for the loss of the expected perfect child. Complex ambivalent or frankly hostile feelings, which may have been present during pregnancy, become significant. Following the birth of a normal child, these negative feelings are usually forgotten, but, if the child is defective, the ambivalent feelings and hostile fantasies may be remembered and thought to be in some way causal (Vernon, 1979).

Parents may blame themselves for acts or omissions or project such blame on to others, particularly professionals. For example, the father of a child born with a facial cleft was convinced that this had been caused by the fingers of the midwife examining his wife during the labour.

Parents of a visibly different child face additional and more specific stresses. Disfigurement involving the face is a serious challenge to a parent's feelings about his or her own worth, competence and image (Lax, 1972). The problem can never be hidden, confronting the mother every time she attends to the baby. Carter (1993), the mother of a baby with an extensive port wine stain has observed, 'The birthmark took over to the extent where the child was *the condition* and the rest of the healthy baby remained invisible' (Carter, 1993). When newborn babies are taken out the face is often the only part visible and their appearance may be the only possible point of conversation.

Professionals' management of such traumatic events has been shown to have a major influence on the ability of the family to cope with the child's condition (Burton, 1975). Staff, shocked like the parents, often freeze initially and feel uncertain about what to say or do. Such behaviour is unhelpful to parents, who can be gently assisted out of their own paralysis by seeing others handle and interact normally with their baby.

The way in which parents are told of the diagnosis, and the emotional impact of this, also have long-term implications for future care. Studies have shown that dissatisfaction with hearing such news is not inevitable (Cunningham and Sloper, 1977). Several arrangements are appreciated by parents: first, being told the diagnosis as soon as possible with their partner present: second, being told directly but sympathetically, in private and with access to the baby: third, opportunity for several subsequent interviews soon after the initial telling so that further questions can be asked.

Uncertainty and delays in diagnosis are stressful to parents, especially if they have felt that professionals have been dismissive of their fears. A frequent example is reassurance that the baby's unusual head shape is due to moulding during birth. With rare conditions, professional ignorance, if not frankly admitted, can allow personal prejudice to intervene. Professionals are certainly not immune to the stereotypes widely held in society regarding physical appearance. A common experience for parents of a facially disfigured baby is to be told that their child will be learning disabled. If this proves to be inaccurate, parental trust in professionals is diminished, even though the outcome is better than predicted.

Attachment

Attachment, first to the child's main care-giver, and later to other important individuals, is basic to the emotional security of us all (Bowlby, 1969). If the attachment develops optimally in the early years, the infant becomes securely attached and is then able to face the rest of the world in a confident manner. If this is not achieved, the infant becomes anxiously (or insecurely) attached, showing either a pattern of anger, being difficult to comfort and excessively distressed by short separations: (anxious/ambivalent pattern), or showing unusually little stress on separation, with avoidance of the mother when reunited: (anxious/avoidant pattern).

Various features suggest that facially disfigured infants are at higher risk than those of normal appearance of developing an insecure attachment, particularly of the anxious/avoidant pattern. The main determinant of secure attachment appears to be the mother's sensitivity and responsiveness to her infant (Crittenden and Ainsworth, 1989). From the time of birth, a mother may be less available to her facially disfigured baby. At two days old, less attractive babies are held less close and given less ventral contact than infants seen as attractive (Langlois and Sawin, 1981). Mothers may also be 'shocked' by the child. Such withholding of physical contact is a powerful determinant of anxious/avoidant attachment. Parents infer emotional states from the child's facial expression, but craniofacial deformities, particularly those affecting the normal movement of the mouth and eyes, may result in misinterpretation. The mother then fails to respond appropriately to the child's needs. Such lack of sensitivity affects the developing attachment. The mother's failure to respond also results in a decrease in the rate of infant smiling so that opportunities for reciprocity and mutually satisfying social interaction diminish (Gewirtz, 1965). For all these reasons facially disfigured children may be at greater risk of insecure attachment than normal children, although this is certainly not inevitable.

We can infer the quality of the attachment by closely observing the mother–child interaction. Studies have looked in detail at aspects of early parenting using video recordings of free interaction and structured situations, which are then rated on predetermined variables. A drawback in such research with facially disfigured children is the impossibility of the rater being 'blind' to the child's condition in controlled studies. Methodological problems with small numbers and a mixture of diagnoses, some of which are associated with additional problems such as feeding difficulties and speech delay, make the identification of significant variables difficult.

Field and Vega-Lahr's study (1984) of mothers and their infants with cleft lip and palate found the mothers to be less active during interaction than mothers of infants with a normal appearance. Wasserman and Allen (1985) compared the interaction of mothers and a) children with either facial or orthopaedic deformities b) premature children and c) healthy two year olds (Wasserman and Allen, 1985). At 24 months, the mothers of the facially disfigured children were significantly more likely to ignore their children than were mothers in other groups.

Barden et al. (1989) studied mothers with craniofacially deformed children and mothers with infants of normal appearance, observing them at four months of age. The mothers of deformed infants behaved in a consistently less nurturant manner than mothers of children without disfigurement. The mothers themselves were unaware of these difficulties, rating their satisfaction with parenting more positively on self-report measures than did the mothers of normal appearance infants.

These studies incline to the view that facially disfigured children experience less sensitive, less responsive and less nurturant parenting from their mothers than do infants of normal appearance and that this impaired interaction is of a kind that may prejudice the development of secure attachment.

For most children, a failure to develop secure attachment will affect their future emotional well-being and interpersonal functioning. For a few, this situation will be even more drastic. If parents fail to begin to cope, then lack of responsiveness may become overt neglect or rejection and it appears that children with facial anomalies are more likely than those of normal appearance to be fostered, adopted or placed on the Child Protection Register. There is, therefore, the potential for the consequences of poor quality mother–child interaction to be devastating. This makes it essential for early identification of such problems. Early intervention to promote a more positive style of interaction can ameliorate a situation which is both unrewarding for the mother and fails to provide the infant with an emotionally nurturing environment.

Siblings

A disabled or chronically ill child in a family is highly stressful for all family members. Parents' time is disproportionately directed to the disabled child, family resources are stretched and healthy siblings may be expected to assume more responsibility at home than their peers. Children may also suffer from the increased stress on their parents, which is associated with higher levels of marital conflict (Speltz et al., 1990).

Methodological weaknesses may account for the variation in findings of the effects on siblings but there are some significant influences. Socioeconomic status, birth order and age gap, the gender of the disabled child and the sibling, and the type of disability, are all relevant. The range and severity of psychological problems is greater in the physically healthy siblings of disfigured children than in those with 'hidden' conditions (Lavigne and Ryan, 1979). Three reasons are suggested. The siblings are discriminated against socially, being stigmatized by their association with the visibly different child. Secondly, the healthy siblings may undergo a change in perception of their own body image, resulting in a change in their behaviour, particularly if they are twins. Clinical experience suggests that a child of normal appearance with a facially disfigured twin often has more psychopathology than the child with the disfigurement, especially if they are 'identical'. Additionally, parents may become overprotective of all their children when disfigurement follows an accident which can make the unaffected siblings irritable and frustrated.

As with facially disfigured children, the siblings' problems do not correlate with the severity of the condition reinforcing the view that the unpredictability of social responses to milder conditions may cause more stress to the child and siblings than a severe condition where negative responses are expected (Lansdown et al., 1991). Younger siblings may be more at risk than older children because of the higher number of adjustments they need to make to cope with changed circumstances, such as alternative care arrangements during hospitalization of the disfigured child.

Generally, the problems for siblings decrease as they become older and develop a life outside the family, but further difficulties emerge during the mid-teens when they start developing relationships with the opposite sex. Young people may become ashamed of their facially disfigured sibling and be reluctant to invite new friends home. Evidence suggests that stigmatization by association operates in this context, as potential partners are apprehensive about the genetic implications of having a facially disfigured child in the family.

Siblings of disfigured children may be reluctant to express their concerns, feeling guilty about apparently complaining when their problems seem less obvious than those of the disfigured child. Addressing such concerns as a family, with professional help if necessary, assists in promoting more openness about the feelings and needs of individuals and acknowledges the impact of facial disfigurement on all family members.

Developmental and maturational issues

No single characteristic or personality type has been shown by research to be associated with specific syndromes or facial disfigurements in general (Clifford, 1983). Those working clinically in the field see children who are seriously troubled by their facial appearance but who show this in subtle ways (e.g. by covering their faces when meeting strangers, hiding behind their parents, drawing themselves as monsters, etc.) (McGregor, 1978).

Predictions for the development of facially disfigured children are therefore difficult. However their problems and limitations must be recognized so that they may be offered appropriate intervention. The important role played by attractiveness in development has been well described by Hildebrandt (1982).

Physical development

General physical development is not affected by facial disfigurement unless there are associated structural anomalies of the palate, airways, etc. which may affect growth due to feeding or breathing difficulties. Failure to thrive may also be a reflection of neglect or inadequate emotional nurturing, and, once physical problems are excluded, psychosocial assessment is necessary with particular attention to the quality of the mother–child interaction. Hearing and speech problems are common and, in some syndromes, there may be visual impairment.

Psychosocial development

Anxiety in disfigured children is more common than in children of normal appearance, especially in social situations (Pertschuk and Whitaker, 1987). Social withdrawal is frequent and avoidance of the stress associated with meeting others further undermines confidence. Greater dependence on significant adults and depression in adolescence have been reported (Lefebvre and Munro, 1978; Pillemer and Cook, 1989).

Self-esteem is a rather poorly defined concept and its measurement is problematic. Most studies have shown the facially disfigured to be in the normal range of self-esteem or even higher (Lefebvre *et al.*, 1986) with others reporting it to be impaired (Lefebvre and Munro, 1978; Pertschuk and Whitaker, 1987). Leonard *et al.*'s study (1991) of children and adolescents with cleft lip and palate found that adolescent girls had a more negative self-concept than younger girls, and adolescent boys had a more positive self-concept than younger boys, although almost all were within the normal range (Leonard *et al.*, 1991). Lefebvre *et al.* (1986) also noticed a sharp decrease in self-confidence during the teens in young people with Apert's syndrome (Lefebvre *et al.*, 1986). It appears that facially disfigured children, especially girls, gradually internalize the negative inferences they experience in social interaction, even if their temperament in early childhood has been reasonably robust.

Behaviour problems are less well studied. Speltz *et al.* (1993) found more behaviour problems reported by both parents and teachers at school entry than in children generally and linked them to poor mother–child interaction observed in infancy. A small number of older children exhibit conduct problems of a disruptive and unco-operative nature. They appear to be inviting negative responses from adults for their behaviour, which they can control, rather than for their appearance, which they cannot. Adolescents may engage in acting out behaviours such as delinquency, and drug and alcohol misuse because of their poor self-esteem and their need to seek solace and peer group acceptance.

Intellectual development

School age children with facial clefts have been shown to score at significantly lower levels than normal children on standardized tests of achievement and on parents' and teachers' ratings of achievements. After leaving school they earn less than their unaffected siblings, again suggesting underachievement. Tests of intelligence have been inconclusive with some claims that children with clefts have significantly lower IQs (Richman and Eliason, 1982).

Some children with facial disfigurement due to congenital syndromes or chromosomal anomalies have specific conditions known to be associated with a high risk of intellectual impairment, but there are few conditions in which this can be predicted with certainty. For example, Apert's syndrome has a very variable impact, with a range of intellectual functioning from average to severe learning disability (Patton *et al.*, 1988).

Schooling

School experiences have a considerable influence on children's development. The sudden increase in the number of strangers the child encounters provides a vast potential for uncertain or negative social responses. The size of the school and the community to which the child belongs is important, and any change of school will increase anxiety.

Teachers' expectations of pupils' academic achievements have been shown to be influenced by physical appearance, with more attractive children being regarded as cleverer, more likely to achieve and more likely to possess positive temperamental characteristics (Dion *et al.*, 1972). As a result, facially disfigured children may be inadequately stimulated or be deprived of specialist resources. Their work is marked less favourably, their misdemeanours punished more harshly, and they receive less of the teacher's attention.

Attractiveness is also a major influence on peer relationships. Children notice disfigurement in early childhood and, from as early as three years of age, preschool children show a significant preference for choosing more attractive peers as friends (Conant and Budoff, 1983). Unattractive children are thought to behave in a more antisocial way and are less likely to be afforded positive qualities such as kindliness, friendliness, happiness, etc. by peers (Dion and Berscheid, 1974). In a study where children were asked to choose friends from drawings of disabled children, the children showed a strong tendency to stigmatize the child with a minor facial disfigurement.

Children portrayed as having a range of significant physical handicaps were preferred as potential friends with only an obese child being rated even less favourably than the facially disfigured child (Sigelman *et al.*, 1986). Facially disfigured children have smaller peer groups which tend to decrease further as the child moves into adolescence. Isolation and stigmatization make facially disfigured children frequent targets of teasing, bullying and ridicule. The differential treatment by teachers and peers may reinforce each other's attitude to the facially disfigured child, so compounding the child's difficulties.

Teaching disfigured children communication skills, boosting their self-esteem and educating teachers and other pupils about the nature and consequences of facial disfigurement are all important in promoting a positive school experience.

Adolescence

Forming new relationships is difficult for the facially disfigured adolescent because their confidence in social relationships has been steadily eroded. Without a wide peer group, they lack the opportunities to try out new relationships and experiences. Even those with a wide circle of same-gender friends complain that they are ignored by the opposite sex.

Leaving school presents a further major social challenge with the need to seek work and attend interviews. Facially disfigured adolescents are inevitably disadvantaged when seeking work as potential employers harbour all the prejudices previously described and are reluctant for facially disfigured employees to have contact with the public. The aspirations of young people with facial deformities are lower than those with conditions which may be more likely to affect performance but are 'invisible' (Goldberg, 1974). Social skills training and appropriate career advice may help disfigured young people at this important stage in their lives.

Surgery

Surgery is very significant for most facially disfigured children and their families. From the moment the problem is identified, parents are anxious to know what can be done to improve their child's appearance and when this can be carried out. Many are anxious for early surgery before the child faces the challenge of starting school, but many factors, such as growth, psychosocial functioning, the nature of the condition and the child's physical state must all be considered when deciding on the nature and timing of any intervention.

Although plastic surgeons may make incredible improvements to children's appearances, society often expects the impossible in the form of a completely 'normal' face. Failure to achieve this has led to parents being criticized for not obtaining appropriate help for their children. Another common anxiety for parents is a fear that surgery will change their children to the extent that they are unrecognizable. They anticipate a child, who postoperatively, is a stranger, both physically and in terms of personality.

At the same time, they fear losing the child they know and love just as they are. Such problems are usually short-lived and as the facial swelling subsides after surgery over the course of a few days, parents gradually recognize their child as fundamentally unchanged, although with an improved facial appearance. For parents who have had major difficulty coming to terms with their child's deformity, surgery may be seen in terms of a rebirth and an opportunity to start building an improved relationship. This is facilitated by professionals dealing with the family around the time of surgery being sensitive to the extent of the difficulties parents may have had.

Conclusion

Facial disfigurement is a constant and continuing source of stress and disadvantage for children and their families. From the time the deformity is first evident, which may be as early as the antenatal period if picked up on an ultrasound scan, the child is at risk of stigmatization and rejection. While some children show remarkable resilience in combating such adversity, evidence supports the view that the majority will have a degree of impairment in their psychosocial functioning and development which specifically relates to their abnormal facial appearance.

The child's family is included by association in society's stereotyping and negative view of such conditions, and this, combined with the additional stress of coping with a special needs child, has important implications for each individual member and for the functioning of the family as a whole.

References

Barden, R. C., Ford, M. E., Jensen, A. G., et al. (1989). Effects of craniofacial deformity in infancy on the quality of mother–infant interactions. Child Dev., **60**, 819–824.

Bowlby, J. (1969). Attachment and Loss. New York: Basic Books.

Burton, L. (1975). The Family Life of Sick Children. London: Routledge & Kegan Paul.

Carter, R. (1993). Personal view: a good colour. Br. Med. J., **307**, 1365.

Cash, T. F., Gillen, P and Burns, S. D. (1977). Sexism and beautyism in personnel consultant decision making. J. Appl. Psychol., **62**, 301–307.

Clifford, E. (1983). Why are they so normal? Cleft Palate J., **20**, 83–84.

Conant, S. and Budoff, M. (1983). Patterns of awareness of children's understanding of disabilities. Ment. Retard., **21**, 119–125.

Crittenden, P. M. and Ainsworth, M. D. S. (1989). Child maltreatment and attachment theory. In Child Maltreatment: theory and research on the causes and consequences of child abuse and neglect (Cicchetti and Carlson, eds.), pp. 432–463, Cambridge: Cambridge University Press.

Cunningham, C. and Sloper, T. (1977). Parents of Down's syndrome babies: their early needs. Child Care Health Dev., **3**, 325–347.

Dion, K. K., Berscheid, E. and Walster, E. (1972). What is beautiful is good. J. Pers. Soc. Psychol., **24**, 285–290.

Dion, K. K. and Berscheid, E. (1972). Physical attractiveness and peer perception among children. Sociometry, **37**(1), 1–12.

Field, T. and Vega-Lahr, N. (1984). Early interactions between infants with craniofacial anomalies and their mothers. Infant Behav. Dev., **7**, 527–530.

Gewirtz, J. L. (1965). The cause of infant smiling in four child-rearing environments in Israel. In Determinants of infant behaviour, vol. 3 (B. M. Foss, ed.) London: Methuen.

Goldberg, R. T. (1974). Adjustment of children with invisible and visible handicaps – congenital heart disease and facial burns. *J. Counselling Psychol.*, **21**, 428–432.

Hildebrandt, K. A. (1982). The role of physical appearance in infant and child development. In *Theory and Research in Behavioural Paediatrics*, vol. 1 (H. E. Fitzgerald, B. M. Lester and M. W. Yogman, eds.), pp. 181–219, New York: Plenum.

Langlois, J. H. and Sawin, D. B. (1981). Infant physical attractiveness as an elicitor of differential parenting behaviours. Paper presented at The Society for Research in Child Development, Boston.

Lansdown, R., Lloyd, J. and Hunter, J. (1991). Facial deformity in childhood: severity and psychological adjustment. *Child Care Health Dev.*, **17**, 165–171.

Lavigne, J. V. and Ryan, M. (1979). Psychological adjustment of siblings of children with chronic illness. *Pediatrics*, **63**, 616–626.

Lax, R. (1972). Some aspects of the interaction between mother and impaired child: mother's narcissistic trauma. *Int. J. Psychoanal.*, **53**, 339–343.

Lefebvre, A. and Munro, I. (1978). The role of psychiatry in a craniofacial team. *Plast. Reconstr. Surg.*, **61**, 564–569.

Lefebvre, A., Travis, F., Arndt, E. M. and Munro, I. R. (1986). A psychiatric profile before and after reconstructive surgery in children with Apert's syndrome. *Br. J. Plast. Surg.*, **39**, 510–513.

Leonard, B. J., Brust, J. D., Abrahams, G. and Sielaff, B. (1991). Self-concept of children and adolescents with cleft lip and/or palate. *Cleft Palate Craniofac. J.*, **28**, 347–353.

McGregor, F. C. (1978). Ear deformities: social and psychological implications. *Clin. Plast. Surg.*, **5**, 347–350.

Patton, M. A., Goodship, J., Hayward, R. and Lansdown, R. (1988). Intellectual development in Apert's syndrome: a long term follow up of 29 patients. *J. Med. Genet.*, **25**, 164–167.

Pertschuk, M. J. and Whitaker, L. A. (1987). Psychosocial considerations in craniofacial deformity. *Clin. Plast. Surg.*, **14**, 163–168.

Pillemer, F. G. and Cook, K. V. (1989). The psychosocial adjustment of pediatric craniofacial patients after surgery. *Cleft Palate J.*, **26**, 201–208.

Richman, L. C. and Eliason, M. (1982). Psychological characteristics of children with cleft lip and palate: intellectual, achievement, behavioural and personality variables. *Cleft Palate J.*, **19**, 249–257.

Sigelman, C. K., Miller, T. E. and Whitworth, L. A. (1986). The early development of stigmatizing reactions to physical differences. *J. Appl. Dev. Psychol.*, **7**, 17–32.

Solnit, A. and Stark, M. H. (1962). Mourning and the birth of a defective child. *Psychoanal. Stud. Child*, **16**, 9–24.

Speltz, M. L., Armsden, G. C. and Clarren, S. S. (1990). Effects of craniofacial birth defects on maternal functioning postinfancy. *J. Pediatr. Psychol.*, **15**, 482–489.

Speltz, M. L., Morton, K., Goodell, E. W. and Clarren, S. K. (1993). Psychological functioning of children with craniofacial anomalies and their mothers: follow up from late infancy to school entry. *Cleft Palate Craniofac. J.*, **30**, 482–489.

Vernon, M. (1979). Parental reactions to birth-defective children. *Postgrad. Med.*, **65**, 183–190.

Wasserman, G. and Allen, R. (1985). Maternal withdrawal from handicapped toddlers. *J. Child Psychol. Psychiatry*, **26**, 381–387.

Chapter 18

Individual variation in adjusting to visible differences

Tim Moss

Introduction

This section of the book considers individual differences in the psychosocial consequences of 'abnormal' appearance – that is, why some people find it difficult to cope and other people manage to adjust more easily. Research concerned with individual differences clearly has important implications for treatment, both medical and psychological. Within this section, discussion of 'abnormal' appearance should be taken to refer to *perceived* abnormal appearance.

An examination of the literature on the implications of disfigurement reveals that being visibly different can be associated with serious psychosocial adjustment problems. It is also clear that the most intuitively obvious features which may influence adjustment, the severity and visibility of the disfigurement, are not strong predictors. Severity has been shown not to be the major predictor of adjustment in maxillofacial patients (Sykes, Curtis, and Cantor, 1972), burn patients (Knudson-Cooper, 1981; Tarnowski *et al.*, 1991) and children with a cleft lip/palate (Landsdown *et al.*, 1991). A similar pattern of equivocal findings exists when the visibility of the disfigurement is considered. It is therefore necessary to consider psychological factors which may play a more crucial role.

Coping

One of the factors which may influence the adjustment of disfigured people is the way they cope with the situations they find stressful. Not all methods of coping are helpful, and successful coping relies on the use of several strategies, at different times. Coping can be cognitive (the way people think about situations), and behavioural (the things people do).

Lazarus (1993) and Carver *et al.* (1989) have produced thorough reviews of coping. The kind of strategies they discuss cover an initially daunting range of methods, including confronting or distancing oneself from risk, self control, seeking social support for either emotional reasons or practical advice, accepting responsibility, planful problem solving, reappraisal, suppression of competing activities, use of religion, venting emotions, and mental or behavioural disengagement. Rather than explain and discuss the utility of each of these strategies separately, it makes sense to categorize them into two broad groups.

We can distinguish between 'emotion-focused coping' and 'problem-focused coping'. The former requires people either to change the way they attend to the threat (for example, by denying it's existence, or concentrating fully on it) or to change the meaning of the threat (for example, thinking, 'That person is staring at me because they are surprised.' instead of 'That person is staring at me because they think I am ugly.'). The common element here is that the way the person thinks and feels about the threat has changed, rather than the threat itself. Problem-focused coping, on the other hand, involves doing something that will change the threat itself (confronting the person who is teasing, getting help or advice to deal with it). Typically, in situations in which it is possible for the person to exercise control over the stressful event, problem-focused coping is effective. In situations in which the stressor is not directly controllable by the person, emotion-focused coping is most effective. One way of helping people adjust is to assist them in identifying the elements of difficult situations over which they can exercise control. This picture is, of course, a simplification. Any stressful event will be best coped with using a combination of coping strategies before, during, and after the event, and the adaptive value of any particular strategy depends upon the context in which it is used.

Keeping the broad distinction between emotion- and problem-focused coping in mind, it is valuable to now consider more specific categories of coping strategy.

Social support

Rumsey and Robinson (in Chapters 15 and 16) discuss the effects of social support on visibly different people. Although equivocal, the evidence is largely supportive of the beneficial effects of social support. What remains to be investigated is why some people seem able to make better use of it than others, and how to help those not benefiting from social support maximize what help is available. To do this, the features of social support that are valuable, and the situations in which they are effective must be identified. Five different types of social support can be offered by the professional worker or by family, friends, and colleagues. These are 'cognitive support' (advice, information), 'social sanctioning' (approval/disapproval), 'material help' (financial or practical assistance), 'companionship' (support of doing things with others), and finally, 'emotional support' (providing a shoulder to cry on) (Kleber and Brom, 1992). Each of these types of support has different characteristics, and it is possible to see that they will have different roles in adjustment. A lot of social contact, alone, does not necessarily equate to useful social support. In order to assess whether the social support a person receives is useful, the subjective needs of the person must be compared with the type of support received. It will not be helpful to someone in need of emotional support or companionship, if the 'support' of people around them consists of practical advice and assistance. Once again, psychological evidence has highlighted the importance of perceived control over stressful events; Carver et al. (1989) have demonstrated that practical social support (similar to Kleber and Brom's cognitive and material types of social support), and not emotional social support, tends to be used in situations which are perceived as controllable.

Brewin *et al.* (1989) consider the possibility of low social support as a consequence, as well as a cause, of poor adjustment. In regard to stigmatized individuals (including the disfigured), they argue that it is possible that stigma produces anxiety, which leads to social withdrawal. This then results in low social support availability. This idea is supported by Folkman *et al.* (1986), who found that situations in which self-esteem is threatened (as it is when stigma produces anxiety) are associated with less social support seeking. Brewin *et al.* (1989) have investigated the relationship between cognitive appraisal of events, and perception of the amount of social support available. They found that low consensus judgements (believing that typically, other people do not have to cope with this situation), as well as believing that the event was likely to recur, and that similar stressful events would happen in a variety of circumstances, were associated with a perception of lower amounts of social support available. It follows that those working with stigmatized groups can help by assisting them to identify realistic levels of support, which may have been systematically underestimated.

In summary, studies of social support have indicated that its role in adjustment to 'abnormal' appearance is likely to be not only the level of social support available, but the type of support, and a person's appraisal of the availability of support. Help can be offered by matching the type of support available to the individuals' needs, and identifying sources of support.

Social skills

An area related to the use of social support is the level of social skills possessed by an individual. It has been well demonstrated that good social skills are related to better adjustment in disfigured populations (Kapp-Simon *et al.*, 1992; MacGregor, 1990; Rumsey *et al.*, 1986; Rumsey *et al.*, 1993). The last of these studies has demonstrated prospectively that social skills training can improve adjustment. A well-argued case has been made for a reciprocal relationship between poor social skills and poor adjustment (see, for example, Bull and Rumsey, 1988). People with poor social skills elicit negative reactions from other people. This feedback contributes to a worse self-image and, consequently, they find it even harder to function in a socially skilled way. Self-consciousness, social anxiety, or anticipation of negative reactions from other people, lead them to behave in a less socially skilled way (initiating fewer conversations, making less eye-contact, etc.). Other people interacting with them react both to their unskilled behaviour, and to their appearance. It is their poor social skills that are responsible for much of the negative reaction that they receive from other people, and these negative reactions are significant causes of difficulties in adjustment.

A recent and thorough review of the way people use this type of interpersonal feedback has, however, questioned the assumption that people use feedback from others to develop their self-image (Kenny and DePaulo, 1993). Rather, they claim, the reverse is true – people interpret feedback on the basis of their existing self-image. In actuality, it is most likely that elements of both occur. Self-image is affected by feedback, and feedback is interpreted in line with the expectations built up by the person's self-image. Social skills training may need to be assessed over a longer term to properly assess this reciprocal relationship. While it is valuable to teach improved management of social encounters to disfigured people and to recognize the benefits of this approach, it is also possible to question exactly which elements of social skills training help. It is likely that coping strategies are taught as part of the 'package', both implicitly and explicitly. By understanding at a more fine-grained level which elements of social skills training mediate improvement, and which of them can be reduced to coping strategies, not only will it be possible for social skills training to be oriented towards inclusion of these factors, but people who do not have access to social skills training courses may also be advised.

Optimism

Carver and Scheier (1985) define optimism as a generalized expectancy for a good outcome. There is strong evidence that this trait is associated with good physical and mental health (e.g. Carver and Gaines, 1987; Scheier *et al.*, 1989). There is evidence that optimism and pessimism predict distress related to surgery for breast cancer, up to 12 months postoperatively (Carver *et al.*, 1993). It is reasonable to predict that a disfigured patient appearing positive about the future, and expecting a good outcome, is more likely to adjust well. It is important however, to realize that the association between optimism and positive outcomes does not mean that optimism *causes* the good results. It is more likely that optimism reflects peoples understanding of their own coping abilities. Unless these underlying abilities are changed, increasing someone's optimism would not bring about a resulting improvement in their adjustment. Several studies demonstrate that this is the case; optimists behave and think differently when faced with threatening circumstances (e.g. Aspinwall and Taylor, 1992). More specifically, they tend to think actively about, and attempt to deal with, difficulties rather than denying them or giving up.

The findings of a beneficial effect of optimism, mediated by coping methods, are strongest in studies where people can realistically use their knowledge of how they have coped in comparable situations in the past. The studies which have found evidence associating optimism with better outcome are those which have examined generalized stressful circumstances, such as life transition, or dealing with a self-selected recent stressful event. Unusual circumstances, where previous coping tactics may not be relevant (e.g. Stanton and Snider, 1993) have not demonstrated the beneficial effects of optimism. This suggests that while optimism can be a predictor of better adjustment, this is more likely if awareness of one's own ability to cope is relevant to the stressful circumstances encountered. This may implicate 'self-efficacy' (Bandura, 1977) as a further underlying factor. The term *self-efficacy* relates to the belief about one's ability to successfully achieve a goal, given actual or observed previous experience of the task. Optimism is less specific, and relates to beliefs about positive outcomes across a variety of situations, whether or not there has been any experience to base this belief on. People with high self-efficacy beliefs, across a number of different types of situations may be mistakenly considered optimistic. Rather than optimism, these people would be basing their expectation of success on previous evidence of their own performance or that of others. The discrepancy between the apparent beneficial effects of optimism in familiar circumstances, and neutral effects in unfamiliar circumstances is thus explained.

In practical terms, this means that rather than simply encouraging a belief that 'things will turn out alright', people coming to terms with 'abnormal' appearance can be helped best by assistance with the development of self-efficacy beliefs. This means helping them to recognize situations in which they have managed well in the past, and helping them to develop transferable skills with which to be able to tackle new situations.

Social comparison

A theory of social comparison was proposed originally by Festinger (1954), and has since been somewhat elaborated. Essentially, social comparison is a technique which some people employ to reduce their sense of being a victim. The theory has specifically included stigmatized groups, such as the disfigured, during its development. In discussing the problems of adjusting to 'abnormal' appearance, a professional worker should be able to identify spontaneous social comparisons. Taylor *et al.* (1983) identified five different types of social comparison. The first of these, downward comparison, has received the most attention. This involves comparison between the self and a person who is even more of a victim than the self, along relevant the dimension (such as appearance).

For example, a person may quote specific examples of people who have had similar experiences to themselves, but have fared worse ('My accident may have left me scarred, but at least I didn't end up looking like she did!').

Other forms of social comparison are comparison along different dimensions (for example, age – 'I may have a scarred face, but it is not as bad for me as for someone in their teens'), creation of hypothetical worse worlds ('I may have lost part of my face through cancer, but I am lucky that it didn't kill me.'), finding meaning from the event ('The way I look may cause me problems, but I have learned what is important in life.'), and invention of a normative level of adjustment, which the person can exceed ('Yes, I am a victim, but I am managing very well.').

As with all coping strategies, the above methods are not equally effective in all circumstances. Recent research has suggested that for downward social comparison at least, people who benefit most have low self-esteem, and are experiencing the threat of victimization (Aspinwall and Taylor, 1993). If social comparison is to be incorporated into treatment, it follows that any intervention will be most effective when coinciding with periods of low self-esteem or victimization. When using social comparisons in treatment, it will not necessarily be helpful to suggest specific comparisons – they should arise spontaneously. However, inviting people to think about possible unspecified comparisons may produce spontaneous, and beneficial comparison.

Denial and avoidance

In certain circumstances, denial and avoidance can be an adaptive form of emotion-focused coping. For uncontrollable events, where there is no effective action which a person could take, denial/avoidance may be more effective than focusing on the threat. Focusing on the threat can have the counter-productive result of increasing distress, without producing any relief. It is potentially beneficial, for example, to be able to deny that one is being stared at by strangers in the street, as there is nothing one can do to stop it. There is some evidence that denial is more useful as a short-term coping strategy (Levine *et al.*, 1987). If this was the case, situations which pass fairly quickly, such as a stranger's glance, would be better coped with by denial than longer-term stressors, such as repeated questioning by a close friend. Maintaining denial becomes more difficult over time, as evidence against the position which the 'denier' is attempting to maintain (that the stressor does not exist) continues. Additionally, there is evidence to suggest that at least some of the benefits of denial arise by providing the person breathing space to marshal other coping resources (Davey, 1993).

In some situations, however, denial may prevent a person finding behavioural solutions to situations which need action to prevent deterioration (for example, denying the symptoms of a chronic illness is not helpful if it prevents people taking action which could improve their prognoses). It has also been claimed that it prevents people properly integrating the event into their 'self-system' (the way they understand themselves and their own experiences) (Roth and Cohen, 1986).

Understanding that denial can be beneficial in some circumstances has practical repercussions. It is not always best to make people 'face up to' their difficulties, unless it is clear that there are alternatives which would be better, and the denial is not preventing an improvement in adjustment. If people are getting benefit from denying that negative events exist in their lives, and this is not doing harm, there is no good reason to discourage them.

Attributions

One way in which people give meaning to events is through the use of causal attributions. Certain styles of explaining negative events have been associated with depressed mood, and poor emotional adjustment – particularly explaining the cause of an event as global (applicable across a range of situations), stable over time, and internal (caused by oneself, rather than someone/thing else). In particular, lonely and shy people tend to use this type of attributional style to account for interpersonal failures (Anderson *et al.*, 1983).

When the attributions of people who are stigmatized, or who are visibly different, are examined, it is clear that biases exist in the way they make attributions about the cause of their difficulties. Essentially, stigmatized people tend to attribute the negative behaviour of other people to the stigmatizing condition, often incorrectly. Crocker *et al.* (1991) investigated the stigmatizing effects of race in attributions about negative feedback. In a controlled experiment, they found that Black Americans over-attributed negative feedback to racial prejudice. They hypothesized that this bias serves to protect the self-esteem of a stigmatized group. In the case of those stigmatized by 'abnormal' appearance, similar attributional errors also arise. Kleck and Strenta (1980) found that subjects in an experiment who were led to believe that they had a false facial scar visible to others (when in fact, the false scar had been surreptitiously removed) attributed much of an interactant's behaviour to prejudice due to their 'abnormal' appearance. McArthur (1982) found that being 'physically distinctive' is associated with more internal attributions for negative social events. In summary, then, those stigmatized by 'abnormal' appearance are at risk of over-attributing the negative behaviour of other people to their 'abnormal' appearance. This over-emphasis on the effects of their appearance can distort the ability of disfigured people to recognize alternative explanations for events. By blaming their appearance, they are relinquishing their ability to change the course of negative social situations, and to engage in problem-focused coping strategies. However, it is also true that, as Crocker *et al.* (1991) point out, these attributions have a self-serving function; by blaming other peoples' prejudice about their appearance for negative social events, disfigured people are able to maintain their self-esteem.

In an examination of self-blame, a difference has also been revealed between characterological and behavioural self-blame (Janoff-Bulman, 1979). In the former, a failure is blamed on a personality trait or characteristic, rather than a specific behaviour. Of these two, characterological self-blame is associated with more negative consequences than behavioural self-blame (Anderson, 1983). If disfigured people blame a social failure upon their 'abnormal' appearance (which is analogous to characterological self-blame), rather than the way they deal with someone's reaction to the way they look (behavioural) more negative emotional consequences would ensue. Tangey *et al.* (1992) note the similarity between characterological self-blame, described above, and the affect of shame, associated with stigmatized groups. Shame has been described as central to the emotional response to stigma (Goffman, 1968). Characterological self-blame is associated with more shameful affect than behavioural self-blame. In other words, people with 'abnormal' appearance who blame their difficulties upon their appearance, rather than their behaviour, are likely to feel more ashamed of themselves. Recent developments in theories of shame (e.g. Gilbert *et al.*, 1994) promise to be very relevant to the problems of emotional adjustment to 'abnormal' appearance.

PTSD

A further potential reason why some people may adapt well, and others badly, is the presence of post-traumatic stress disorder (PTSD) in some disfigured people. PTSD is an anxiety disorder recognized by five diagnostic criteria: first, having experienced a markedly distressing event; second, persistent recollection of the event (in bad dreams, similar events, etc.); third, persistent avoidance of things associated with the event; fourth, increased arousal (sleeping difficulties, irritability, etc.); and finally, presence of these signs for at least a month after the trauma. PTSD has been observed most notably in war veterans, rape victims, and disaster victims. It has also been observed in burn victims (Perry *et al.*, 1992; Williams and Griffiths, 1991). In the Perry *et al.* study, up to 40 per cent of burn patients had developed PTSD when assessed six months after the burn. The predictors of whether an individual would develop the disorder were social support, area of body surface burned, and the initial level of emotional distress. Interestingly, the severity of disfigurement associated with the burn was not a predictor of PTSD development. A recent article has suggested that the concept of PTSD could be extended beyond circumstances following a particular traumatic event. Scott and Stradling (1994) suggest that similar symptomatology can be observed in people who have undergone prolonged duress – hence, prolonged duress stress disorder (PDSD). This is even more applicable to the daily problems encountered by people with disfigurements. It is important to recognize that people with disfigurements may be suffering from PTSD/PDSD as a result of either a traumatic cause of the disfigurement, or the repeatedly stressful social consequences of the disfigurement. Unlike PTSD, the concept of PDSD has not yet received widespread support, and future developments will be observed with interest by those with an interest in adjustment to stigmatizing conditions. If people have been avoiding situations which bring to mind the traumatic events associated with the disfigurement, have difficulty thinking about other things, and have sleeping difficulties/nightmares, they may be suffering from PTSD/PDSD, rather than more general adjustment problems, and need specialist attention.

Conclusions

There is no simple model to explain why some people adjust well, and others poorly, to comparable problems of appearance. The clearest conclusion to emerge from an examination of individual differences is that it is the way people think about situations which governs both their emotional and behavioural reactions to them. Without addressing the way people interpret what is happening in their lives – be it through appraisal associated with coping, perceptions of self-efficacy, social comparison, attributional style etc. – interventions risk missing the mark. It is apparent though, that there is a wealth of relevant psychological theory which has rarely been used in properly constructed empirical studies of adjustment. As this theoretical background becomes more fully developed in relation to the practical problems of coping with abnormalities of appearance, better intervention strategies can be developed and treatments can be planned around patients' needs and strengths.

References

Anderson, L.G. (1983). Motivational and performance deficits in interpersonal settings: the effect of attributional style. *J. Pers. Social Psych.*, **45**, 1136–1147.

Anderson, C.A., Horowitz, L.M. and French, R. (1983). Attributional style of lonely and depressed people. *J. Pers. Social Psych.*, **45**, 127–136.

Aspinwall, L.G. and Taylor, S.E. (1992). Modelling cognitive adaption: a longitudinal investigation of the impact of individual differences and coping on college adjustment and performance. *J. Pers. Social Psych.,* **63**(6), 989–1003.

Aspinwall, L.G. and Taylor, S.E. (1993). Effects of social comparison direction, threat, and self esteem on affect, self-evaluation, and expected success. *J. Pers. Social Psych.,* **64**(5), 708–722.

Bandura, A. (1977). Self-efficacy: towards a unifying view of behavioral change. *Psych. Rev.,* **84**, 191–215.

Brewin, C.R., MacCarthy, B. and Furnham, A. (1989). Social support in the face of adversity: the role of cognitive appraisal. *J. Res. Pers.,* **23**, 354–372.

Bull, R. and Rumsey, N. (1988). *The Social Psychology of Facial Appearance.* New York: Springer Verlag.

Crocker, J., Voelkl, K., Testa, M. *et al.* (1991). Social stigma: the affective consequences of attributional ambiguity. *J. Pers. Social Psych.,* **60**(2), 218–228.

Carver, C.S. and Gaines, J.G. (1987). Optimism, pessimism, and post-partum depression. *Cogn. Ther. Res.,* **11**, 449–462.

Carver, C.S., Pozo, C., Harris *et al.* (1993). How coping mediates the effect of optimism on distress: a study of women with early stage breast cancer. *J. Pers. Social Psych.,* **65**(2), 375–390.

Carver, C.S., Scheier, M.F. (1985). Self-consciousness, expectancies, and the coping process. In *Stresses and Coping* (T. Field, P.M. McCabe and N. Schneiderman, eds.), pp. 305–330. Hillsdale, NJ: Erlbaum.

Carver, C.S., Scheier, M.F. and Weintraub J.K. (1989). Assessing coping strategies: a theoretically based approach. *J. Pers. Social Psych.,* **56**, 267–283.

Davey, G.C.L. (1993). A comparison of three cognitive appraisal strategies: the role of threat devaluation in problem-focused coping. *Pers. Individual Diff.,* **14**(4), 535–546.

Festinger, L. (1954). A theory of social comparison processes. *Hum. Relat.,* **7**, 117–140.

Folkman, S., Lazarus, R.S., Dunkel-Schetter, C. (1986). Dynamics of a stressful encounter: cognitive appraisal, coping, and encounter outcomes. *J. Pers. Social Psych.,* **50**, 992–1003.

Gilbert, P., Pehl, J. and Allan, S. (1994). The phenomenology of guilt and shame: an empirical investigation. *Br. J. Med. Psych.,* **67**, 23–36.

Goffman, E. (1968). *Stigma.* London: Penguin Books.

Janoff-Bulman, R. (1979). Characterological versus behavioural self-blame: inquiries into depression and rape. *J. Pers. Social Psych.,* **37**, 1798–1809.

Kapp-Simon, K.A., Simon, D.J. and Kristovich, S. (1992). Self-perception, social skills, adjustment and inhibition in young adolescents with craniofacial anomalies. *Cleft Palate – Craniofac. J.,* **29**(4), 352–356.

Kenny, D.A. and DePaulo, B.M. (1993). Do people know how others view them? An empirical and theoretical account. *Psych. Bull.,* **114**(1), 145–161.

Kleber, R.J. and Brom, D. (1992). *Coping With Trauma: Theory, Prevention, and Treatment.* Amsterdam: Swets and Zeitlinger.

Kleck, R.E. and Strenta, A. (1980). Perceptions of the impact of negatively valued physical characteristics on social interaction. *J. Pers. Social Psych.,* **16**, 348–361.

Knudson-Cooper, M.S. (1981). Adjustment to visible stigma, the case of the severely burned child. *Soc. Sci. Med.,* **15**, 31–44.

Landsdown, R., Lloyd, J. and Hunter, J. (1991). Facial deformity in childhood: severity and psychological adjustment. *Child: Care, Health, and Dev.,* **17**, 165–171.

Lazarus, R.S. (1993). Coping theory and research: past, present and future. *Psychosom. Med.,* **55**, 234–247.

Levine, J., Warrenburg, S., Kerns, *et al.* (1987). The role of denial in recovery from coronary heart disease. *Psychosom. Med.,* **49**, 109–117.

MacGregor, F. C. (1990). Facial disfigurement: problems and management of social interaction and implications for mental health. *Aest. Plast. Surg.,* **14**, 249–257.

McArthur, L.E. (1982). Physical distinctiveness and self-attribution. *Pers. Social Psych. Bull.,* **8**(3), 460–467.

Perry, S., Difede, J., Musngi, G., (1992). Predictors of post traumatic stress disorder after burn injury. *Am. J. Psychiatry,* **149**(7), 931–935.

Roth, S. and Cohen, L.J. (1986). Approach, avoidance and coping with stress. *Am. Psychologist,* **41**(7), 813–819.

Rumsey, N., Bull, R. and Gahagen, D. (1986). A developmental study of childrens' stereotyping of facially deformed adults. *Br. J. Psych.,* **77**, 269–274.

Rumsey, N., Robinson, E. and Partridge, J. (1993). *An Evaluation of The Impact of Social Skills Training for Facially Disfigured People.* Bristol: Changing Faces.

Scheier, M.F., Matthews, K.A., Owens, *et al.* (1989). Dispositional optimism and recovery from coronary artery bypass surgery: the beneficial effects on physical and psychological well-being. *J. Pers. Social Psych.,* **57**, 1024–1040.

Scott, M.J. and Stradling, G.S. (1994). Post-traumatic stress disorder without the trauma. *Br. J. Clin. Psych.,* **33**, 71–74.

Stanton, A.L. and Snider, P.R. (1993). Coping with breast cancer diagnosis: a prospective study. *Health Psych.,* **12**, 16–23.

Sykes, B.E., Curtis, T.A. and Cantor, R. (1972). Psychosocial aspects of maxillofacial rehabilitation, Part II. A long range evaluation. *J. Prosthetic Dentistry,* **28**, 540–545.

Tarnowski, K.J., Rasnake, L.K., Gavaghan-Jones, M.P., *et al.* (1991). Psychosocial sequelae of pediatric burn injuries: a review. *Clin. Psych. Rev.,* **11**, 371–398.

Tangey, J.P., Wagner, P. and Gramzow, R. (1992). Proneness to shame, proneness to guilt, and psychopathology. *J. Abnormal Psych.,* **101**(3), 469–478.

Taylor, S.E., Wood, J.V. and Lichtman, R.R. (1983). It could be worse: selective evaluation as a response to victimisation. *J. Social Issues,* **39**(2), 19–40.

Williams, E. and Griffiths, T. (1991). Psychological consequences of burn injury. *Burns,* **17**(6), 478–480.

Chapter 19

Assessment and measurement in clinical practice

Tony Carr

Adults

The nature and purpose of assessment

The effectiveness of the care and treatment we offer to patients depends upon the extent to which the strategies we use actually meet the patients' needs. The choice of a treatment strategy, therefore, involves a judgement that the preferred treatment is more likely to meet the needs of the patient than are alternative treatments. This central process of clinical judgement is one of matching probable treatment outcomes to patients' needs and is dependent upon good knowledge of both. Consideration of the technical merit of a treatment clearly is a matter of professional judgement. Equally clearly, the value of particular clinical outcomes rests upon patients' judgements about the extent to which these outcomes actually meet their needs. Good clinical care therefore requires adequate knowledge of the patient's needs as well as information about the likely success of a treatment in meeting those needs for a particular patient.

In clinical practice, assessment is the means by which we can identify and measure the extent of the patient's needs. Appropriate assessment also provides important information about the personal and social resources, and limitations, which people bring with them into treatment and which are likely to interact with treatment in determining a more or less successful outcome. In a very real sense, there is never any treatment without prior assessment although, all too often, the assessment is peremptory, routine or narrow and is not designed to address the full range of the patient's potential needs. Effective assessment rests upon clinicians having a clear picture of what they need to know in order to make informed decisions about care and treatment: it is only when the objectives of assessment are clear that we can decide what issues we need to explore, what we need to assess and what methods to use.

What should we assess?

A sound basic principle is to ensure that prior to any assessment we are clear about what we need to know and what method or strategy we are planning to use to obtain the information we need. However brief, extensive, structured or unstructured the interaction with the patient, the most useful assessments are planned around a number of broad questions, the answers to which will inform our decisions about patient care (e.g. How much difficulty does this person experience in social situations? How disturbed is her sexual relationship? How much of her difficulty does she attribute to her disfigurement?). Such broad questions may constitute a written checklist to guide an extensive assessment or may simply be explicit questions 'in our heads' as we pause momentarily in preparation for a brief interaction with a patient on a ward round or in the day room.

Although the information we need may change as the patient moves from initial assessment, through treatment to discharge and follow-up, there is sufficient research evidence about the difficulties experienced by people with disfigurements (e.g. Harris, 1982; and see Chapters 15, 16 and 18) for us to identify the main areas for assessment. These areas of investigation are set out in Figure 19.1: the list is not exhaustive and does not cover physical assessment nor assessment of the disfigurement (for the latter see Chapters 14 and 20). The methods by which these areas may be assessed are discussed below.

1. Current difficulties
   Social interaction: meeting people, attending social events
   Public exposure: shopping, travelling, walking in the street
   work, school/college
   Leisure: hobbies, activities and interests
   At home: domestic tasks, answering the door, garden/outside activities
   Relationships: family, friends, colleagues, marriage, sex
   Self-care: eating, sleeping, washing, shaving, make-up, dressing/ undressing
2. Current state
   Usual emotional state and present emotional state: anxiety, depression, sadness, irritability, self-consciousness, shame, anger, embarrassment
   Self-concept: self-liking/disliking, self-worth, good/bad, strong/ weak
   Specific coping strategies: dress, hair, camouflage, posture, avoidance, withdrawal, assertiveness
   Attributions: which difficulties are attributed to the disfigurement
   Quality of life
   Anticipations of treatment outcome, motivation
   Concerns about the future: events of personal significance which may be adversely affected by existing dysfunctions or by aspects of treatment and/or recovery
3. Stable factors
   Usual coping style: successful/unsuccessful, emotion-focused/ problem-focused, optimistic/pessimistic, resilience, determination, courage

Attributional style: internal/external
Social support: availability, ability to use
Interpersonal style: warmth/coolness, humour, social skills
Educational level, verbal fluency, employment, housing, finances

4. Historical and developmental issues
    Where difficulties associated with the disfigurement predate the assessment, useful insights may be gained by exploring their development, particularly through an investigation of their onset and subsequent course in terms of the 'who', 'what', 'when', and 'where' of significant events.

Figure 19.1

Assessment methods

In broad terms there is an unavoidable trade-off in assessment methods between flexibility and accuracy. The more flexible and sensitive a method is, the more subject it is to bias, distortion and omission: the less subject it is to bias and distortion, the less flexible it is in use. The two extremes of this flexibility/accuracy dimension are unstructured clinical interviews (very flexible but highly subject to distortion) and standardized psychometric tests and inventories (very resistant to distortion but deliberately focused and inflexible).

The choice of assessment method is a matter of matching the method to the task. Interviews will be used to answer broad questions such as 'what type of problems does this patient experience?', where flexibility and sensitivity are required to explore the patient's life and to respond to his immediate needs for support etc. Standardized tests and inventories are used when the questions are more specific, e.g. 'How anxious is this patient?' or 'What social difficulties does he experience and how frequently?'. Of course, there are also clinical situations where the use of a standardized scale would be insensitive and inappropriate and there are areas of investigation for which no appropriate scales are available. In such situations verbal strategies are necessary, despite their susceptibility to distortion, and we need to take what steps we can to minimize unreliability and bias.

The clinical interview

Whatever form the interview takes, it is most effective when carried out against a background of rapport with the patient. Without a degree of rapport it is unlikely that patients will feel able to reveal or discuss matters that are sensitive, or about which they feel shame or anticipate ridicule and rejection. Throughout the interaction, the clinician needs to be self-aware and to purposefully express sincerity, acceptance, understanding, genuine interest and a positive regard for the worth of the person. Research has shown that rapport is built most effectively on the patient's perception of the interviewer's warmth, genuineness, empathy, unconditional positive regard and perceived competence (Truax and Carkhuff, 1965). Clearly, these attributes are conveyed verbally, non-verbally and behaviourally, and may be improved by practice with feedback. Detailed guidelines on the development of rapport and the use of non-verbal behaviour are beyond the scope of this chapter, but many excellent expositions exist (e.g. Egan, 1986; Truax and Carkhuff, 1965).

As discussed earlier, the main strength of the interview as a method of assessment lies in its flexibility. This flexibility gives the clinician freedom in the order in which topics are addressed, the depth to which issues are explored and opportunities for verification or clarification of information provided by the patient. This allows the interview to be conducted in a way that is maximally responsive to the patient's needs at the time and which, therefore, conveys acceptance, understanding, interest and empathy.

An assessment of a disfigured patient could be based upon the topic areas set out in Figure 19.1. For a full assessment, all the areas listed would need to be covered at some point in the interview. For a briefer assessment, such as a postoperative or follow-up assessment, an appropriate selection from this larger list would need to be made according to prior knowledge of the patient. Clearly, each topic area will need to be converted into a series of questions, with open questions predominating early on in the interview and more direct questions being used later to fill in gaps in information and to confirm details (Maloney and Ward, 1976). The basic skills of open-ended questioning, continuing statements, clarifying, probing and summarizing are fundamental to effective interviewing and are well described elsewhere (e.g. Egan, 1986).

The dangers of unreliability, error and omission in interviews are ever-present as the 'price' asked for flexibility. Numerous studies have shown that the agreement between interviewers using unstructured interviews (expressed as a correlation) is highly variable, typically ranging from .23 to .97 with a median value of .57 (Arvey and Trumbo, 1965; Wagner, 1949). Of particular relevance is the extent to which different interviewers focus on different areas and how this can be counteracted and reliability improved when topic areas are specified and training is provided (e.g. Dougherty *et al.*, 1986). The implication for clinical practice is the value of structuring the content of the interview, at least to the extent of using a checklist of the areas to be covered. Such a checklist obviously guards against omissions and minimizes the bias of interviewers.

Interviewer bias is a significant threat to the validity of interviews. For example halo effects can lead an interviewer to assume other supposedly related attributes having once formed a general impression of a patient. For example, patients who express warmth interpersonally may be seen as more competent or healthy than they actually are. These associations may be incorrect and can lead to error or distortion. Physical attractiveness has been shown to produce positive interviewer bias (Gilmore *et al.*, 1986) and first impressions have been found to bias later judgements (Cooper, 1981). Research on the accuracy of clinical judgements indicates that it is not associated with age, females are slightly better than males on average, and it is positively associated with higher intelligence, artistic/dramatic interests, good emotional adjustment and similarity in race and cultural background (Shapiro and Penrod, 1986; Vernon, 1964). A final caution, especially for experienced interviewers, is that confidence in clinical judgements has often been shown to be unrelated to the accuracy of those judgements (e.g. Lichtenstein and Fischoff, 1977; Oskamp, 1965).

In summary, the clinical interview offers an approach to assessment which can be responsive to circumstance, to the needs of individual patients and to the uniqueness of patients' experience. However, as a source of information, it is highly susceptible to error through omission, bias and distortion. The practical question is how to minimize the sources of error while retaining the strengths of the interview. Perhaps the most important step is to structure the field of enquiry by constructing a checklist based upon the topics in Figure 19.1. Flexibility can be maintained by not following these in a rigid order but, nevertheless, ensuring that all are covered by the end of the interview, and that any unusual aspects of the patient's experience have been adequately explored.

The use of summarizing at points throughout the session, where the clinician's understanding is 'offered' for the patient's confirmation, is a valuable defence against error and assumption. Assumptive biases are also minimized by a determined avoidance of closed questions, for example, 'Do you feel upset when that happens?', and a reliance upon open questions such as 'How do you feel when that happens?'. An awareness of the influence of halo effects and the interviewer's own biases and assumptions, together with a deliberate attempt to explore possibilities in the patient's account which run counter to expectations, also helps to increase validity and reliability. With these precautions, the clinical interview is an indispensable method of assessment but, in view of its susceptibility to error, information gleaned on critical issues should be corroborated by other methods whenever this is possible. Potential alternative methods of assessment which are more specific and focused than the clinical interview are considered later in this chapter.

Brief encounters of the verbal kind

As an approach to assessment, short discussions with patients are susceptible to the same sources of error as clinical interviews. However, they are typically much more focused and benefit from the corroborative effect of greater depth and detail in a limited area of enquiry. In a brief encounter it is important to establish effective rapport quickly and to 'set the agenda' early. In practical terms, the use of accurate empathy (see Egan, 1986) and the removal of obvious obstacles to communication are the first steps. In this context, typical obstacles are standing at the bedside of prone patients rather than getting down to the patient's level for good eye contact, overlooking the patient's need for privacy when discussing sensitive or distressing issues and expecting patients in a state of undress to relate comfortably to a professional who is fully clothed.

The importance of 'setting the agenda', that is explaining what we want to discuss, is that in the absence of an explanation patients will always make their own assumptions about the purpose of the interaction. When the patient's perceived purpose differs from the actual intent of the discussion communication difficulties such as defensiveness, evasion and misunderstanding frequently result. With care short, well focused discussions are valuable opportunities for obtaining information, especially when the patient and clinician are already familiar with each other and trust has been previously established.

Observational methods

The obvious limitation of interviews is that they depend entirely upon patients' perceptions and recollections of events and experiences. This makes all information obtained in this way subject to the vagaries of memory and the many factors which produce error and distortion in recall. Ideally, interview data should be bolstered by methods of assessment which are less subject to memory effects: these include observation *in vivo* (in real life), observation during role-play and self-monitoring. *In vivo* and role-play observation are not normally practicable in routine clinical settings but are a central feature of psychological assessments in the areas of interpersonal and social problems which are the most pertinent to the care and treatment of disfigured patients (Bellack and Hersen, 1988; Spence, 1994). Self-monitoring, which uses patients as their own observers, takes advantage of the fact that the patient is the only person present in every relevant event and all such events take place *in vivo*.

Self-monitoring can be used to obtain further, detailed information on any issue identified in interview. Provided not too much is asked in terms of recording, it is practicable with most patients. The key to successful self-monitoring is to obtain the patient's co-operation in recording a small number of well-defined, specific events. The events to be recorded may be occurrences in the usual sense, such as talking with strangers, or they may be emotions, such as feelings of embarrassment. With occurrences, patients may be asked simply to record their frequency each day over a period such as two weeks, or they may be asked to record more detail (e.g. time, place, setting, people present, what happened, feelings experienced and who did what before during and after the specified occurrence). With emotions such as embarrassment, anxiety and anger it is important to include in the record the thoughts that accompany the emotion, since the event with which the emotion is associated may be in the past or the future. To minimize problems of recall, it is important to encourage patients to complete the record as frequently as possible during each day. It is usual for self-monitoring data obtained in this way to give a much clearer picture of the patient's difficulties and, frequently, to provide new insights into the causes of those difficulties.

Not surprisingly, difficulties in compliance may increase in proportion to the complexity of the task. However, patients typically are well motivated in relation to their difficulties and, provided the task is clearly explained and the events well defined, they are usually capable of providing the information requested. The main drawback to self-monitoring as a method of assessment is that it is reactive. That is, it may actually produce changes in the events to be recorded (Kazdin, 1974; Nelson, 1977) and patients may have difficulty with the accurate observation of their own behaviour or may selectively attend to negative aspects of events (Roth and Rehm, 1980). However, the few studies which have investigated the validity of self-monitoring records are consistent in supporting its validity (e.g. Royce and Arkowitz, 1978; Twentyman and McFall, 1975).

Visual analogue scales

Visual analogue scales (VAS) represent one step further in the assessment of patients' experience or behaviour beyond the event recording, obtained in unrefined self-monitoring described above. The VAS offers a simple and practical approach to quantification of the patient's experience. Typically it consists of a horizontal line of fixed length, usually 100 mm, with anchors such as 'completely relaxed' and 'total panic' at the ends, with no labelling of intermediate positions on the line. Respondents are required to mark the line at a point corresponding to their perceived state. With careful choice of unambiguous anchor descriptions, the VAS can be used to measure the patient's experience on any dimension of interest at any time. For example, if we wished to know how obvious patients believe their disfigurements to be to other people we could use 'never detectable by others' and 'always obvious to others' as anchors, and 'not at all embarrassed' and 'overcome with embarrassment' if we wished to know how embarrassed patients felt in certain situations. VASs may be used on their own or may be included in the self-monitoring record.

Most people can complete a VAS without difficulty, but about seven per cent find them problematic and older patients may find a vertical line easier (Huskisson, 1974; Streiner and Norman, 1991). The main problem with VASs is that they are relatively unreliable by virtue of their use of a single dimension, because there is a direct relationship between reliability and the number of items used in a scale of measurement. Strictly speaking, so-called adjectival scales, in which the undivided line of the VAS is labelled with three or five intermediate points, should be used in preference to the VAS to achieve greater reliability. However, this is a more complex undertaking and obviates the simplicity of the VAS, which is its main advantage. The simple VAS is adequate for most purposes. It has many enthusiastic adherents and is widely used in health research and clinical assessment (Bowling, 1991; Streiner and Norman, 1991).

Psychometric scales

By virtue of the rigour with which they are constructed, psychometric scales stand at the opposite end of the error/distortion continuum from the clinical interview. They are constructed to have known characteristics of standardization, reliability and validity which minimize their susceptibility to error and distortion. A good psychometric scale should give very similar results when used by different assessors or when used with the same patient on different occasions (reliability); it should measure all important aspects of the variable(s) of interest; it should measure what it purports to measure (validity); where appropriate, it should have adequate norms which enable the patient's results to be compared with those of comparable groups of patients and others (standardization).

In the context of clinical assessment, psychometric scales are best regarded as a supplement to the clinical interview, to obtain valid and reliable information on important issues already identified, rather than as a substitute for the clinical interview. They can also be used to screen patients, to assess changes in patients pre- and postoperatively and to follow-up patients postoperatively. They are available in a range of formats – observer-rating scales, assessor-administered and self-rating scales, although it is the self-rating format which is most commonly used in health assessment. Unless scales have been specifically designed to be comprehensive (e.g. the General Health Questionnaire and The Derriford Appearance Scale), psychometric scales have a specific focus and a limited range of applicability (e.g. measures of anxiety, depression or pain). There are literally thousands of scales of potential relevance and the interested reader is referred to standard reference works and reviews (e.g. Bowling, 1991) and to the catalogues of test publishers such as NFER and The Psychological Corporation (these catalogues also indicate which scales are restricted and which are available for general use). We shall consider a limited range of scales of particular relevance to assessment in the care of people who are visibly different.

Psychological well-being

The Hospital Anxiety and Depression Scale (HAD) is particularly valuable for use with patients who may be physically unwell since it was designed to give scores which are independent of somatic symptoms (Zigmond and Snaith, 1983). It is a brief assessment of anxiety and depression, consisting of 14 items divided between the two subscales, in which the patient rates each item on a four-point scale (0-3). Typical items are 'I feel tense or wound up', 'worrying thoughts go through my mind' and 'I feel as if I am slowed down'. Criterion scores are given for the presence of depression and anxiety of clinical significance. To date, the evidence for reliability and validity of the scale is reasonable but more work is needed to improve confidence in its psychometric properties.

The General Health Questionnaire (GHQ) is the most widely used measure of psychological disturbance in the UK. Although developed in England (Goldberg, 1978; Goldberg and Williams, 1988) it has also been used successfully in many other cultures and has been translated into about 40 languages. It is a pure state measure, assessing present state in relation to usual state, and provides scores on depression, anxiety, somatic signs and everyday functioning. Although not designed to detect long-standing conditions, very few such cases are missed and a revised scoring method can be used to make the scale more sensitive to chronic conditions (Goodchild and Jones, 1985). The GHQ is available in a number of forms (60, 30, 20, 28, 12 items) of which the GHQ28 is probably the most useful clinically, being brief and providing scores on the four dimensions. Typical items are 'Have you recently felt that life isn't worth living?', 'Have you recently been able to concentrate on whatever you're doing?' or 'Have you recently spent much time chatting with people?'. The scale has been extensively standardized and criterion scores are provided for the identification of people who may be at risk of significant anxiety or depression. Validity and reliability data are good and detailed manuals and user handbooks are available (Goldberg and Williams, 1988). The GHQ is a useful population screening instrument and can be used to monitor change effectively, especially when the revised scoring is used.

Social Performance and Social Anxiety

In the context of disfigurement, the assessment of anxiety and performance in interpersonal and social situations may be of particular relevance and there is a range of self-report measures available. The Social-Situation Questionnaire (SSQ) (Bryant and Trower, 1974; Trower *et al*., 1978) provides self-ratings of both the frequency and difficulty of performing a selection of social behaviours. It is reported to be useful with non-clinical and clinical samples and is sensitive to change following intervention. In the area of interpersonal effectiveness, the Rathus Assertiveness Scale (Rathus, 1973) is the most widely used and well established scale. It has good psychometric properties and a simplified version (McCormick, 1984) has been used with a variety of clinical groups. Among assessment scales for social anxiety, the Social Avoidance and Distress (SAD) scale and the Fear of Negative Evaluation (FNE) scale (Watson and Friend, 1969) are two widely used measures of established reliability and validity. The first assesses the respondent's propensity to avoid and to experience distress in social situations, and the second reflects fears of negative evaluation by others. The two scales may be used together to produce a combined score reflecting social and interpersonal difficulties overall. Although widely used, the SAD and FNE scales were developed on college students and it is preferable, when working with patient groups, to use scales that have been standardized on relevant clinical populations.

Recent developments that meet the criterion of clinical standardization, and which maintain the distinction between anxiety arising from social interaction and anxiety caused by being observed by others, are the Social Interaction Anxiety Scale (SIAS) and the Social Phobia Scale (SPS) (Heimberg *et al*., 1992; Mattick and Clarke, 1989). These companion scales are relatively brief, self-report instruments of 20 items each, rated on five-point response scales from nought (not at all characteristic or true of me) to four (extremely characteristic or true of me). The SIAS items are self-statements describing one's typical emotional, cognitive or behavioural reaction to a variety of situations involving social interaction in pairs or groups and the SPS items cover situations which involve one's actions being observed by others. The scales are standardized on relevant clinical groups (socially anxious and socially phobic) with comparative data for agoraphobic groups and community samples. Heimberg *et al*. (1992) report acceptable reliability and validity for the scales with clinical groups, good differentiation between patients and non-patients and sensitivity to therapeutic change.

Quality of life and life satisfaction

The Affect Balance Scale is an indicator of happiness or general well-being (Bradburn, 1969). It is based upon the hypothesis that subjective well-being can be represented as a person's position on the two independent dimensions of positive and negative affect (feelings). Well-being is expressed as the balance between scores on these dimensions. This combined score allows positive feelings to compensate for negative ones, which is the main strength of the scale. It is a usefully brief scale, with each dimension being represented by five items such as 'on top of the world because someone complimented you', 'things going your way', 'very lonely, remote from people' and 'upset because someone criticized you', with the respondent simply indicating yes or no. Psychometric evaluation shows the scale to have acceptable levels of reliability and validity. It is sensitive to change and can be used with older people.

A more recent and flexible scale for the assessment of general well-being is the Positive and Negative Affect Scale (PANAS) developed by Watson et al. (1988). Like the Affect Balance Scale, it is predicated upon the existence of the two independent dimensions of positive and negative affect and comprises ten affective descriptors for each dimension to which the respondent is asked to indicate on a five-point scale 'to what extent you have felt this way during the past week'. The time base of the scale can be varied according to the time-frame of interest from 'at the present moment' to 'how you feel on average'. In each time-frame, the PANAS has good psychometric properties. It is brief, acceptable and easy to use and, if required, can be substituted for longer, specific measures of anxiety and depression with which it correlates well. The standardization samples are large but, as yet, there is relatively little data on clinical groups. However, the indications are that the scale will perform as well in clinical settings as it does with non-clinical groups.

If there is a need for a scale which is very simple to use, the Delighted-Terrible Faces (DT) Scale may be used. It is brief, readily understandable and can be tailored to any area of the patient's life that is of interest. It consists of seven schematic faces set out in a horizontal line, ranging from A (delighted) to G (terrible) in facial expression, and respondents are asked to indicate which of the faces come closest to expressing how they feel about the specified issue (e.g. life in general, relationships with other people, your appearance). Initial investigations of reliability and validity (Andrews and Withey, 1976) were satisfactory and the scale has been used with a variety of patients and non-clinical samples (e.g. Anderson, 1988; Bowling and Brown, 1991). More work is needed on the psychometric properties of the scale but, at present, its main strength is its ease of use and acceptability to patients.

Clinical Audit

The general need for measures of quality of life to support clinical audit within the NHS has generated a substantial amount of development in relevant methods of assessment. There are two instruments which have been well standardized on British populations – the Nottingham Health Profile (NHP) and the UKSF36. The latter is the most suitable for use with less severely ill or dysfunctional patients for the assessment of quality of life and is available in a number of shorter forms. Both scales are well reviewed by Jenkinson et al. (1993) to which the interested reader is referred. Wood and Tarer (1994) report the development of the Cambridge classification, as a very brief and practicable approach to the routine collection of audit information in plastic surgery. However, at present this is an insensitive measure which is based upon clinicians' judgements and for which there is no reliability or validity data. Cole et al. (1994) specifically address the measurement of quality of life in clinical audit using the Health Measurement Questionnaire (HMQ). This is a brief self-report scale which correlates positively with the NHP and HAD but, for which, there is no reliability data. Cole *et al.* demonstrate its use in deriving quality adjusted life-years (QALYS) but the calculations are not straightforward and more psychometric development is needed before it can be used with confidence.

The assessment of therapeutic outcome in clinical audit by quality of life measures may well be too general and lacks the specificity that can be obtained with the use of a measure of distress and dysfunction in problems of appearance (see below).

Distress and dysfunction in disfigurement

Until recently there have been no psychometric scales for the assessment of emotion and behaviour in people with problems of appearance. The need has been for a single measure which provides a detailed, yet comprehensive picture of the emotional and behavioural difficulties experienced by people whose abnormalities of appearance range from the objectively gross to the aesthetic (see Chapter 14).

The Derriford Appearance Scale (DAS) has been developed to provide a psychometrically sound instrument for clinical and research use in disfigurement (Carr and Harris, 1992; Harris, Carr and Nicholas, 1994). It is available in a long and a short form, both of which have undergone extensive psychometric evaluation. In addition to total scores reflecting overall distress and dysfunction in disorders of appearance, the long form also gives factorial scores on self-consciousness of appearance (covering feelings of unattractiveness, embarrassment, and inferiority, distress from being teased, stared at and talked about and lack of self-confidence), sexual and marital dysfunction, social avoidance and isolation and occupational dysfunction.

The authors report excellent reliability, good validity and sensitivity to clinical change (Harris, Carr and Nicholas, 1995). The DAS is widely acceptable to patients and clinicians and has been constructed to function effectively with all degrees of abnormalities of appearance from normal (non-clinical), through aesthetic to gross disfigurements. Although not yet published, the scale is in the final stages of development and is currently available from the authors who are keen to see it used widely for the generation of an extensive normative data base which will facilitate its use in the assessment of the full range of disfigurements.

Body Dysmorphic Disorder (BDD) and Psychiatric Diagnosis

In the clinical assessment of people with problems of appearance, particularly if their disfigurements are at the aesthetic end of the continuum (Harris, this volume), it can be useful to identify those patients who may be suffering from, or liable to, a psychiatric disorder. It has been argued that the presence of a psychiatric disorder in problems of appearance reduces the likelihood of a successful therapeutic outcome (Phillips *et al.*, 1993). However, it is important to note that this caution applies almost exclusively to psychoses and to psychotic delusions. Severe mood and anxiety disorders are common accompaniments to problems of appearance and may be regarded as secondary to those problems and, thus, do not contraindicate therapy.

The criteria for body dysmorphic disorder (DMS IV, 1994) include 'Preoccupation with some imagined defect in appearance in a normal-appearing person. If a slight physical anomaly is present, the person's concern is grossly excessive'. It is also stated that the belief in the physical defect is not of delusional quality and does not occur exclusively during the course of anorexia nervosa or transsexualism. However, there remains significant dispute about the validity of BDD as an independent diagnostic category (e.g. Hollander *et al.*, 1992) in view of the commonalities with other disorders, such as obsessive-compulsive disorders and social phobias. Furthermore, the implied pathology of a diagnosis of BDD is questioned by the results of 'normal' population surveys which reveal high levels of concern and preoccupation with appearance and body image (e.g. Fitts *et al.*, 1989). In addition to doubts about the validity of a diagnosis of BDD, the clinical value of such a diagnosis must also be questioned since it does not appear to predict the application of a specific or effective therapy (Phillips *et al.*, 1993).

Therapeutic decisions are better matched to patients' characteristics and needs, with improved chances of success, on the basis of careful and comprehensive assessment as described earlier, rather than upon the application of descriptive psychiatric nomenclature.

Children and toddlers (Elizabeth Walters)

The problems of visibily different children cannot be predicted by the severity of their condition; a comprehensive assessment is necessary to identify any difficulties and opportunities for intervention. The assessment of children and families covers three broad areas: the child's psychosocial functioning and level of distress; the family's ability to deal with stress and to promote positive coping in their child; and their suitability and motivation for surgery.

There is a tendency for people to avoid talking to disfigured children about their appearance, fearing that it will be too painful, but children are not damaged by evoking distress, providing it is acknowledged with sympathy and sensitivity. There is no arbitrary boundary between assessment and treatment, and a comprehensive assessment should also be therapeutic. The setting should be appropriate to the age of the child and allow for privacy. Parental involvement will depend on the age of the child.

Babies and toddlers

Assessment at this stage involves observation of the parent–child interaction. The level and type of physical contact with the child should be noted, particularly any difficulty in holding the baby ventrally and eye to eye contact. Reciprocity between parents and the infant, and the responsiveness of the parent to the child, are important. Feeding problems should be described in detail and a record made of the baby's birth weight and subsequent growth.

Parents should be asked if they feel comfortable in taking the baby out, and handling staring and questions from strangers. The reaction of siblings and the extended family should be described. The interviewer should be alert to maternal postnatal depression. Any difficulties parents have expressed in coming to terms with the diagnosis should be gently probed and an assessment made of their expectations of future problems and hopes for surgery.

Children

Children should be seen initially with parents, but always allowed an opportunity to be interviewed alone. There is good evidence that even the most sensitive parents do not have complete knowledge of their child's feelings and experiences. Toys, drawing materials and puppets are useful in helping younger children to express their feelings.

Initially, children should be put at ease by some general factual closed questions before addressing their appearance. After questions about the facial features they like and dislike and would change if they could, open questioning is necessary to elicit their beliefs about causation, their thoughts and feelings and to access their inner world. Young children are unused to talking in this way and, although open questions provide the most accurate information, children who are ill at ease may need to be offered alternatives or suggestions such as, 'Some children tell me that . . .'

Children should be asked about their experiences at home, at school and in the community, and their feelings about such events. More severe teasing may come from siblings rather than other children. Details of teasing, name-calling and bullying are necessary, including the extent, the relationship to the perpetrators, any responses they make, and the reaction of adults around them. Children should be asked to describe an example in detail. Situations they avoid, such as looking in mirrors and taking part in school photographs, should be described. It is also important to ask about details of positive experiences, such as the extent and quality of friendships, and participation in and enjoyment of out of school activities. Enquiries should be made about the school experience, whether it is seen as a place of fear and humiliation or safe and enjoyable. Do their teachers like their work? Do other children like their ideas?

Any areas of particular strength should be sought, such as a sense of humour, academic or sporting ability, artistic talent, etc. The attractiveness of the children's dress, their posture, eye contact and body language are all significant in reflecting their self-esteem, but it should be remembered that children respond especially to the nonverbal communication of the interviewer, so that appropriate eye contact from the interviewer to the child and a relaxed manner are essential. For some children, their problems may go beyond emotional upset and distress, and amount to a psychological disorder such as anxiety or depression. This must be recognized and the need for specialist referral considered.

Adolescents

The social skills of the adolescent should be observed and direct enquiries made about peer group activities and support. Concerns about developing relationships with the opposite sex need to be sought and their need for genetic counselling assessed. Academic achievement should be discussed and ambitions for the future explored.

Interviewers should remain morally neutral to any antisocial behaviour reported and show that they are still interested in the adolescent's feelings, concerns, point of view, etc. If there is any hint of depression, high levels of distress or poor self-esteem, the risk of deliberate self-harm and suicide must be assessed by direct questioning. Addressing such difficult topics can alarm the inexperienced, but bringing up the subject is not likely to act as a trigger for such behaviour and missing the opportunity can be disastrous. Acknowledging the extent of their problems and then asking if the severity of their difficulties has ever caused them to think of harming themselves is an acceptable approach for most young people.

Parents and family

Information should be sought from parents to give further insight into the child's functioning within the family. The amount of stress on the parents and the supports available to them are important. Their coping strategies should be explored and strengths identified. Aspects of family functioning are important, especially their affect (sadness, anger, tension) e.g. communication patterns (verbal and nonverbal), and responsiveness and sensitivity to different family members.

Referral to specialist services

Children and adolescents presenting with severe emotional or behavioural problems may need referral for specialist psychological or psychiatric help. This is essential where there is severe depression or suicidal ideation. Specialist therapy is also necessary if the mother–child relationship is a cause for concern. Mental illness identified in a parent, usually maternal depression, may also need specific treatment. Some families may benefit from family therapy if problems for siblings are significant or if the family functioning is seriously deviant.

Referral to a psychologist for psychometric testing is indicated in three circumstances: first, if there is a suspicion of developmental delay, with either generalized or specific learning disabilities; secondly, if discrepancies exist between apparent educational potential and actual achievement; and, thirdly, if neuropsychological deficits are suspected because of large discrepancies in verbal and performance skills, or problems with memory, visuospatial ability or speed in psychomotor tasks. Children having difficulties primarily in school with learning, behaviour or peer group relationships may be helped by the educational psychologist for their area. Conditions involving the palate or tongue may require a speech and language assessment by a speech therapist.

Assessment for surgery

When surgery is being considered solely for cosmetic reasons, surgeons often request assistance over the appropriateness and timing of any operations. In addition to children's distress and psychological functioning, it is important to interview children to ascertain their expectations for improvement, motivation for surgery and fears of painful procedures. Their need for further factual information should be determined and a view formed of their competence to give informed consent.

The parents' reasons for requesting surgery should be discussed, along with their expectations. A common anxiety for parents is that an altered appearance will mean a change in personality. The extent to which the parents have accepted the child's disfigurement is important, as those who have failed in this process often pressurize their child to have early surgery and have unrealistic expectations for improvement in appearance. The parents' ability to discuss proposals with their child in an appropriate way is important. Even more crucial is their ability to be perceptive to their child's wishes, but not to burden the younger child of insufficient understanding with the sole responsibility for decision making.

References

Anderson, R. (1988). The quality of life of stroke patients and their careers. In *Living with Chronic Illness: The Experience of Patients and Their Families* (R. Anderson and M. Bury, eds), pp. 165–183, London: Unwin Hyman.

Andrews, F. M. and Withey, S. B. (1976). *Social Indicators of Well-being: Americans' Perceptions of Life Quality*. New York: Plenum.

Arvey, R. D. and Campion, J. E. (1982). The employment interview: a summary and review of recent research. *Pers. Psychol.*, **35**, 281–322.

Bellack, A. S. and Hersen, M. (1988). *Behavioural Assessment: A Practical Handbook*. Oxford: Pergamon.

Bowling, A. (1991). *Measuring Health*. Milton Keynes: Open University Press.

Bowling, A. and Brown, P. (1991). Social support and emotional well-being among the oldest old living in London. *J. Gerontol.*, **46**, 20–32.

Bradburn, N. M. (1969). *The Structure of Psychological Well-being*. Chicago: Aldine.

Bryant, B. M. and Trower, P. E. (1974). Social difficulty in a student sample. *Br. J. Educ. Psychol.*, **44**, 13–21.

Carr, A. T. and Harris, D. L. (1992). Psychological effects of plastic surgery. Presented to the *Annual Conference of the British Psychological Society*, Brighton.

Cole, R. P., Shakespeare, V., Shakespeare, P. and Hobby, J. A. E. (1994). Measuring outcome in low-priority plastic surgery patients using quality of life indices. *Br. J. Plast. Surg.*, **47**, 117–121.

Cooper, W. H. (1981). Ubiquitous halo. *Psychol. Bull.*, **90**, 218–244.

Diagnostic and Statistical Manual of Mental Disorders, Fourth Edition (DSM IV) (1994). Washington DC: American Psychiatric Association.

Dougherty, T. W., Ebert, R. J. and Callender, J. C. (1986). Policy capturing in the employment interview. *J. Appl. Psychol.*, **71**, 9–15.

Egan, G. (1986). *The Skilled Helper*. Monterey, CA: Brooks/Cole.

Fitts, S. N., Gibson, P. and Redding, C. A. (1989). Body dysmorphic disorder: implications for its validity as a DSM-III-R clinical syndrome. *Psychol. Rep.*, **64**, 655–658.

Gilmore, D. C., Beehr, T. A. and Love, K. G. (1986). Effects of applicant sex, applicant physical attractiveness, and type of job on interview decisions. *J. Occup. Psychol.*, **59**, 103–109.

Goldberg, D. P. (1978). *Manual of the General Health Questionnaire*. Windsor: NFER-Nelson.

Goldberg, D. P. and Williams, P. (1988). *A User's Guide to the General Health Questionnaire*. Windsor: NFER-Nelson.

Goodchild, M. E. and Jones, D. P. (1985). Chronicity and the General Health Questionnaire. *Br. J. Psychiatry*, **146**, 55–61.

Harris, D. L. (1982). The symptomatology of abnormal appearance: an anecdotal survey. *Br. J. Plast. Surg.*, **35**, 312–323.

Heimberg, R. G., Mueller, G. P., Holt, C. S., *et al.* (1992). Assessment of anxiety in social interaction and being observed by others: the social interaction anxiety scale and the social phobia scale. *Behav. Ther.*, **23**, 53–73.

Hollander, E., Neville, D., Frenkel, M., *et al.* (1992). Body dysmorphic disorder: diagnostic issues and related disorders. *Psychosomatics*, **33**, 156–165.

Huskisson, E. C. (1974). Measurement of pain. *Lancet*, **ii**, 1127–1131.

Jenkinson, C., Wright, L. and Coulter, A. (1993). *Quality of Life Measurement in Health Care.* Oxford: Health Services Research Unit, University of Oxford.

Kazdin, A. E. (1974). Reactive self-monitoring: the effects of response desirability, goal-setting and feedback. *J. Consult. Clin. Psychol.*, **42**, 704–716.

Lichtenstein, S. and Fischoff, B. (1977). Do those who know more also know more about how much they know? *Organ. Behav. Human Performance*, **20**, 159–183.

Maloney, M. P. and Ward, M. P. (1976). *Psychological Assessment: A Conceptual Approach.* New York: Oxford University Press.

Mattick, R. P. and Clarke, J. C. (1989). Development and validation of measures of social phobia, scrutiny fear and social interaction anxiety. *J. Consult. Clin. Psychol.*, **56**, 251–260.

McCormick, I. A. (1985). A simple version of the Rathus Assertiveness Schedule. *Behav. Assess.*, **7**, 95–99.

Nelson, R. O. (1977). Methodological issues in assessment via self-monitoring. In *Behavioral Assessment: New Directions in Clinical Psychology* (J. D. Cone and R. P. Hawkins, eds.), pp. 74–86. New York: Brunner/Mazel.

Oskamp, S. (1965). Overconfidence in case-study judgements. *J. Consult. Psychol.*, **29**, 261–265.

Phillips, K. A., McElroy, S. L., Keck, P. E., *et al.* (1993). Body dysmorphic disorder: 30 cases of imagined ugliness. *Am. J. Psychiatry*, **150**, 302–308.

Rathus, S. A. (1973). A 30-item schedule for assessing assertive behavior. *Behav. Ther.*, **4**, 398–406.

Roth, D. and Rehm, L. P. (1980). Relationships among self-monitoring processes, memory, and depression. *Cogn. Ther. Res.*, **4**, 157–159.

Royce, W. S. and Arkowitz, H. (1978). Multimodal evaluation of practice interactions as treatment for social isolation. *J. Consult. Clin. Psychol.*, **46**, 239–245.

Shapiro, P. N. and Penrod, S. (1986). Meta-analysis of facial identification studies. *Psychol. Bull.*, **100**, 139–156.

Spence, S. H. (1994). Interpersonal problems. In *Clinical Adult Psychology* (S. J. E. Lindsay and G. E. Powell, eds.), pp. 229–252, London: Routledge.

Streiner, D. L. and Norman, G. R. (1991). *Health Measurement Scales: A Practical Guide to Their Development and Use.* Oxford: Oxford University Press.

Trower, P., Bryant, B. and Argyle, M. (1978). *Social Skills and Mental Health.* Pittsburgh: University of Pittsburgh Press.

Truax, C. B. and Carkhuff, R. R. (1965). Client and therapist transparency in the psychotherapeutic encounter. *J. Couns. Psychol.*, **12**, 3–9.

Twentyman, C. T. and McFall, R. M. (1975). Behavioral training of social skills in shy males. *J. Consult. Clin. Psychol.*, **43**, 384–395.

Vernon, P. E. (1964). *Personality Assessment: A Critical Survey.* London: Methuen.

Wagner, R. (1949). The employment interview: a critical review. *Pers. Psychol.*, **2**, 17–46.

Watson, D. and Friend, R. (1969). Measurement of social evaluative anxiety. *J. Consult. Clin. Psychol.*, **33**, 448–467.

Watson, D., Clark, L. A. and Tellegen, A. (1988). Development and validation of brief measures of positive and negative affect: the PANAS scales. *J. Pers. Soc. Psychol.*, **54**, 1063–1070.

Wood, S. H. and Tarer, M. N. (1994). Outcome audit in plastic surgery. *Br. J. Plast. Surg.*, **47**, 122–126.

Zigmond, A. S. and Snaith, R. P. (1983). The Hospital Anxiety and Depression Scale. *Acta Psychiatr. Scand.*, **67**, 361–370.

Chapter 20

Anthropometry: the physical measurement of visible differences

Dai Roberts-Harry

Introduction

Anthropometry may be defined as the measurement of the size, weight and proportions of the human or primate body. This chapter will consider why anthropometry is useful in treating various types of disfigurement and the different methods of measurement that are currently available.

Anthropometric measurements are concerned with description, prescription, prediction, evaluation and research.

Description involves comparing the measurements taken from patients with values taken from a normal population. For instance, in a patient with hemifacial microsomia, a condition affecting asymmetrical growth of the face, we would wish to determine the size and proportion of the upper and lower jaws to see where the problem lies. Measurements of these features could then be compared with those derived from normal data to indicate the extent and nature of the problem.

Prescription is concerned with treatment planning such that optimal results can be obtained. For example, if a patient has a poor facial appearance because of a receding chin, this might be caused by a small lower jaw, a large upper jaw or, possibly, a combination of both. Furthermore, the teeth may be unfavourably tipped, exacerbating the problem. Treatment planning would have to consider all these factors and determine what tooth and jaw movements are needed. The precise amount of movement required in the teeth and the hard and soft tissues can be carefully determined from anthropometric measurements; it is in this area that these measurements are of most value.

Prediction is concerned not only with attempting to evaluate the treatment outcome but also in trying to assess the amount and type of growth that a younger patient may have. Growth can dramatically affect the nature of a particular problem, either by improving or worsening it. Clearly, if the clinician is able to determine the amount and direction of residual growth in an individual, this is extremely useful. Unfortunately, this is an imprecise science because, although average values can be added to the existing shape and size, detailed individual prediction is currently not possible. The best that can be achieved is to assume that the individual would experience average growth changes. Obviously, in individuals with atypical growth, this method of adding average increments will not produce accurate information.

Evaluation of changes that have been produced by either growth or treatment can provide valuable information for the clinician. Measurements taken after any treatment has been completed can show how closely the pretreatment aims have been achieved. When the outcome of treatment is to be assessed, a comparison of pre- and post-treatment measurements is needed. In order to do this, reference structures that have not changed during the treatment need to be used and measured to a high degree of accuracy. Although this is applicable to some methods of anthropometry, the location of landmarks has proved hard in some of the more complex three-dimensional methods of measurement. Reference points are also more difficult to locate in growing patients because it is sometimes not always possible to tell whether the changes that occur are due to the treatment the patient has received or whether they have been affected by growth in some way.

Research is clearly important in the treatment of disfigurement. It is necessary to measure treatment outcome in large numbers of patients so that the optimal treatment protocol can be established for different conditions. Comparisons of this nature usually involve comparing groups of patients that have been treated with one technique with those that have been treated by another. Intercentre comparisons are also possible so that the same treatment method used in different places can be evaluated. In some areas of anthropometry, large data sets obtained from normal individuals have been built up. This allows the comparison of various conditions with the population norm and also the outcome of different treatment regimens.

Measurement techniques

Comparison of dimensions obtained in a specific patient requires a baseline from which measurements can be taken. This involves measuring from standard reproducible landmarks. In addition, a uniform method of measurement and standardization of the measuring equipment are needed. The measurement of the body can be done in a number of ways; a full description of all methods is beyond the scope of this chapter. The methods of investigation that will be considered and described are: physical measurements, plain radiographic measurements, computed tomography (CT) scanning, magnetic resonance imaging (MRI), and laser scanning.

Physical measurements

This practice involves using precision anthropometric instruments to measure different parts of the body. The measurements thus obtained can be compared with published normal values, such as those of Tanner and Whitehouse (1973, 1976). To measure standing height, an upright measuring device called a stadiometer is commonly used and scales may be used for measuring weight. A ruler, callipers, and other measuring devices can also be used. Measurements can be taken directly from the individual, or from photographs if highly standardized photography is used by a technique known as photogrammetric anthropometry.

The number of different measurements of the human body is almost limitless and it is impossible for any one individual to memorize them all. Fortunately, standard reference books are available; for example Hall *et al.* (1989), in which many physical dimensions from various sources are published. These measurements are useful in comparing height and weight with a normal value and can be particularly helpful in many deformities, so that the type and extent can be assessed. For example, in patients with ocular hypertelorism (increased interpupillary distance) comparing measurements between the pupils or orbits with published normal values can reveal the extent of the problem and the type and extent of surgery that would be needed to correct it. Similarly, in patients with long or short faces, the facial measurements can be made and compared with normal values (Farkas, 1981). It is important to realize that one should not slavishly attempt to convert an individual into a series of figures and ratios, but that these measurements are simply a guide to the dimensions of the problem and what corrective steps may be needed.

Plain film radiography

Radiographs can be extremely useful for measuring bony structures. Specific bone lengths and asymmetry can be accurately measured, although the positioning of the area under observation is critical. All radiographs are subject to some degree of magnification and this must be taken into account when obtaining measurements. The most widely used form of measurement obtained from plain film radiographs is that of the head, known as cephalometrics. Cephalometrics, or cephalometric radiography, is a technique for orientating radiographs for the purpose of head measurement. It has been widely used in orthodontic treatment planning and maxillofacial surgery. The technique has been used for the comprehensive collection of cephalometric radiographs of many individuals to produce data sets of normal measurements (Broadbent 1975; Bhatia and Leighton, 1993).

Cephalometric radiographs are taken under standardized conditions, using a machine known as a cephalostat. Although there are many different types of cephalometric analysis, they all measure essentially the same four characteristics: skeletal, dentoskeletal, interdental and soft tissue relationships. Skeletal factors assess the position of the jaws relative to the face and to each other. Dentoskeletal factors measure the position of the teeth relative to the jaws. Interdental relationships assess the position between the teeth in the upper and lower jaws. The soft tissues envelop the skeletal and dental structures and their relationship and dimensions can also be assessed (Figure 20.1).

Measurements are usually taken from a reference point or plane, but variations in the position or orientation of these can affect measurements. Computer-aided programs are available that will plan the required movements and provide a simple visual image of the desired result. Recently,

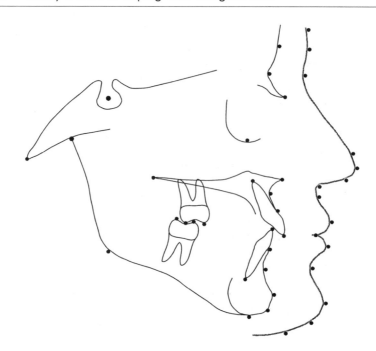

Figure 20.1 A typical outline of a lateral skull radiograph is shown. Some of the commonly used landmarks are indicated by the dots. From these, specific measurements can be obtained to assess various craniofacial dimensions.

computer-aided video capture techniques have been introduced, which will simulate the final facial appearance, although some caution is needed when using these. Whilst it is simple to produce an image of a perfect result on a computer screen it is not quite so easy to do so in practice. Therefore, it is important not to give the patient unrealistic expectations about the benefits of treatment and it is incumbent on the clinician to be pragmatic about the treatment goals.

Computed tomography

Tomograms are images of the body taken with a predetermined thickness or 'slice'. Conventional tomograms are obtained by movement of the X-ray tube and film in opposite directions during exposure. Structures within the plane of interest are sharply defined, whereas those outside this are blurred. Such radiographs produce two-dimensional images. Computed tomography differs from conventional tomograms in that a more sensitive X-ray detection is used, such as gas or crystal detectors, and the data obtained from these are manipulated using a computer. The X-ray tube rotates outside the patient and, in most cases, the exposure is made with a 360° rotation. A three-dimensional image of the area of interest can be constructed and, by moving the patient up and down through the scanner, multiple adjacent sections can be imaged, allowing a picture of the body to be built-up. The slice thickness can be varied; usually it is between 1 mm and 10 mm. The thinner sections provide more detailed information, but greater X-ray exposure is needed.

The data obtained from each set of exposures or slices are reconstructed by computer manipulation to produce a three-dimensional surface image, which can be viewed from any angle on a computer screen. Computed tomographic scanning has clear advantages over plain film radiography in that it shows a three-dimensional image of the body. It illustrates bony and soft tissue structures well. Three-dimensional imaging of this nature is becoming more and more widely used in planning reconstructive and corrective surgery. However, one of the main drawbacks is the high radiation dose needed to visualize accurately a specific part of the body, because of the large number of thin slices that are needed. As a consequence, large data sets have not yet been constructed as has been done for lateral skull cephalometry.

Magnetic resonance imaging

This is a new system of imaging that depends on the magnetic properties of certain tissues. The nuclei of these tissues behave as small magnets and, when placed within a strong magnetic field, will align themselves with respect to that field. Hydrogen ions (protons, in water molecules and lipids) will change their alignment, flipping through a preset angle and then rotate in phase with one another. When the radio-frequency wave is switched off, the protons return to their original alignment. As they do so, a small, but detectable, radio signal is emitted and this is picked up on detection coils placed around the patient. An MRI scanner consists of a large circular magnet within which are radio-frequency transmitter and receiver coils.

The advantage that MRI has over CT scanning is that it will show the soft tissues in greater detail. Calcified tissues do not generate any signal using MRI and may be less precise than a CT scanner at defining the skeletal morphology. However, it produces excellent soft tissue images and can assist the surgeon in planning soft tissue surgery. The considerable advantage that MRI has over CT scanning is that no radiation exposure is needed and there seem to be no long-term adverse affects produced by MRI. However, it is contraindicated at present in patients with certain types of aneurism clips and cardiac pacemakers because of the strong magnetic fields involved. Currently, MRI is a slow process compared with CT scanning, requiring a long scan time of several minutes. The patient must also keep still during the scanning procedure. Although MRI is a relatively new technique, it is already being used for describing abnormalities of soft tissues and planning corrective treatment for facial and limb disfigurement.

Laser scanning

This is a method of three-dimensional image capture, described and developed by Moss et al. (1988). It utilizes a low-power helium neon laser, which is scanned across the patient's face or body. The reflected beam is captured by a video camera and the information analyzed by specially developed software and stored on computer. The image can be reconstructed on a computer screen and rotated in any direction, so that all the individual features can be seen. This system has the advantage over many other types of physical anthropometric measurements in that a large number of points are captured by the laser scanning in a very short time. Typically, 20 000 points are digitized in approximately 15 seconds and the accuracy of the scan has been quoted to be to 0.5 mm by Coombes *et al.* (1991). These authors felt that this method of analysis of facial morphology could form the basis for a quantitative description of the changes in facial appearance following surgery and during growth, and that it will aid the development of normative standards of facial aesthetics.

Summary

The field of anthropometry has advanced a long way from the simple use of rulers and callipers. Particularly in the areas of CT scanning, MRI and laser scanning, new and exciting possibilities are emerging in assessing and planning treatment for patients with disfigurement. Recently Linney *et al.* (1993) described a system that produces a display of anatomical surfaces from CT, MRI and ultrasonography. Displays are created that show the three-dimensional internal and external anatomy of the subject. The images can also be manipulated on the screen and it is possible to plan surgery by simulation. This system can also drive a milling machine for the production of models, prostheses and implants for use during surgical correction.

References

Bhatia, S. and Leighton, B. (1993). *Manual of Facial Growth: A Computer Analysis of Longitudinal Cephalometric Growth Data.* Oxford University Press, Oxford, UK.

Broadbent, B. H., Broadbent, B. H. Jr. and Golden, W. H. (1975). *Bolton Standards of Dentofacial Developmental Growth.* St Louis, MO, Mosby.

Coombes, A. M., Moss, J. P., Linney, A. D., Richards, R. and James, D. R. (1991). A mathematic method for the comparison of three-dimensional changes in the facial surface. *Eur. J. Orthod.*, **13**, 95–110.

Farkas, L. G. (1981). *Anthropometry of the Head and Face in Medicine.* New York: Elsevier.

Hall, J. G., Froster-Iskenius, U. G. and Allanson, J. E. (1989). *Handbook of Normal Physical Measurements.* Oxford: Oxford University Press.

Linney, A. D., Tan, A. C., Richards, R., Gardener, J., Grindrod, S. and Moss, J. P. (1993). Three-dimensional visualisation of data of human anatomy: diagnosis and surgical planning. *J. Audio. Media Med.*, **16**, 4–10.

Moss, J. P., Grindrod, S. R., Linney, A. D., Arridge, S. R. and James, D. (1988). A computer system for the interactive planning and prediction of maxillofacial surgery. *Am. J. Orthod. Dentofac. Orthop.*, **94**, 469–475.

Tanner, J. M. and Whitehouse, R. H. (1973). Height and weight charts from birth to five years allowing for length of gestation. *Arch. Dis. Childhood*, **48**, 786–789.

Tanner, J. M. and Whitehouse, R. H. (1976). Clinical longitudinal standards for height, weight, height velocity, weight velocity and stages of puberty. *Arch. Dis. Childhood*, **51**, 170–179.

Coping with Visible Difference

Edited by Eileen Bradbury

Chapter 21

Introduction to Section Three

Eileen Bradbury

In the first section of this book, the contributors have described their own personal history and daily experience, and the ways in which looking different has affected their lives and those of their families and friends. There is a diversity of experience, but there are common themes that can be identified. These include feelings of loss, adverse social reactions and the interactions with the professionals who have treated them. In the second section, which focused on what has been learned from the literature in this field, wider issues relating to visible difference were discussed. Historical, cultural and social factors that have influenced reactions to disfigurement were explored. Thus, individual responses have been described in the context of a broader academic approach.

From this work it is clear that there are common stresses relating to disfigurement, mediated by individual differences. These stresses have been shown to have a significant impact on the lives of the individuals affected and on their families. What can be done to help? This section looks at ways in which those with visible differences can be helped to cope. This may be through the organization of services, through individual or group counselling, and/or through support groups. Just as there is a wide diversity of individual experience, so there are various ways in which people can find help to develop coping skills.

This book assumes an interest in the subject because of some contact with people with visible differences. The reader may be a nurse working on a burns unit, a liaison sister in plastic surgery, a social worker whose client has been disfigured, a speech and language therapist working with children with clefts, a clinical psychologist involved in issues relating to reconstructive surgery, or one of many other professionals who may find this book useful as a resource. Although there is no assumption of a specific professional background, it is assumed that the reader has at least a rudimentary understanding of counselling. This includes an awareness of issues such as confidentiality, effective listening and an ability to relate to the client in an empathic and nonjudgemental way. The cultural and social context of disfigurement has been described in Section Two; we may all be subject to emotional responses within that context. Reactions such as shock, distress and/or blaming would make it difficult to establish a therapeutic relationship that is the basis of any psychological intervention. A major aim of this section is to offer a guide to a clinical understanding of what needs and can be done, and to allow the reader to incorporate that knowledge into his or her own professional expertise.

This section opens with an account of what is currently available within the National Health Service and how those services are organized, including a discussion of how people can gain access to them. Specific services are described in order to illustrate how they can be run, with a description of the possible pitfalls and the difficulties that can occur. The reality is that provision is patchy. In some areas, and for some conditions, appropriate support is available to the client group, whilst in other areas of the country and for other conditions, the service is either nonexistent or offers little psychological support. The interaction between the medical/surgical professionals and those offering psychological and other therapeutic intervention is described, and the difficulties that can arise are discussed.

Having considered those services that are available, the section then goes on to consider how they can be enhanced through psychological support and intervention with the client. Drawing on the first two sections of this book, consideration is given to broad themes and general psychological and social problems that have been found to be a common experience for many with disfigurement. Following each general problem, there is guidance on how the client can be helped to cope.

There is a limit to how general it is possible to be in this field. Whilst there are common issues for this client group, it is always important to assess and work with individual responses. In order to offer guidelines for this, individual case studies describe how individuals with a particular constellation of problems can be assessed and then helped to cope. These case studies are intended to illustrate specific ways of helping with specific problems in the broader context of visible difference. They are not prescriptive and should not be used as a total package. It is very important that the individual responses are understood and that specific forms of intervention are picked from those described in this book.

These case studies do not describe real individuals, but are created from the authors' clinical experience and are intended to demonstrate typical case histories. Their purpose is to allow more detailed examination and discussion of the issues.

Those with physical differences are often offered treatment such as reconstructive surgery, laser treatment and medication. Some such interventions are essential (e.g. the repair of a cleft palate). However, there are other forms of surgery that are not necessary for the physical well-being of the client, such as improving the appearance of scarring. This requires decisions to be made based on psychological and social, as well as medical issues. The chapter on decision making looks at the factors that need to be taken into account, such as individual need, the competence of a child, expectations about outcome, the timing of surgery, and when enough is enough. The aim of this chapter is to focus on these issues and to help the reader to facilitate stable and competent decision making by adults and children. There is an examination of the implicit factors that might affect that decision making, such as distress and anxiety, and also explicit factors, such as ways of framing questions and information processing.

Working in this field can be stressful, as professionals struggle to cope with their own emotional responses to disfigurement. In Section Two, it has been clearly shown that the impact of disfigurement can be immense for the individual, for the parents of a newborn baby with a visible difference, for the family, and for the casual observer in the street. Professionals working in the field are not immune to such stress and may need support to help them to cope with their own responses. Chapter 26 looks at the issue of professional support and how that can be structured and implemented.

Those with a visible difference may feel that they need contact with others who have the same condition. This can be offered through support groups, and many such groups exist. Chapter 27 looks at the issue of support groups and examines the potential benefits and drawbacks for the individual and for the families of those with disfigurement.

Having considered what the problems can be, what interventions are currently available and how the individual reader can help, the focus then shifts to a consideration of good practice. The final chapter draws from the rest of the book in order to describe ways of providing effective services to meet the needs of those with visible differences. This provides a framework within which intervention can be implemented.

Summary

The aims of this section are:

1. To examine current provision in this field;
2. To give the reader an understanding of the problems of those with a visible difference.

The objectives of this section are:

1. To look at specific types of service provision and examine their strengths and weaknesses;
2. To identify common problems experienced by those with a visible difference;
3. To describe strategies of intervention to help the reader to tackle these problems;
4. To describe in detail interventions for specific situations;
5. To identify ways of offering professional support;
6. To facilitate decision making.

Chapter 22

Psychological intervention and models of current working practice

Daniela Hearst and Judith Middleton

In this chapter we look at the different ways that disfigured people come into contact with help from the National Health Service (NHS), whether in outpatient clinics or as admissions for surgery. The medical, surgical and psychological needs of an individual child or adult can be complex and long lasting; often surgery is undertaken over many years. The patient and their family are, therefore, entering into a long and complicated relationship with the hospital system and with professionals.

There is a common perspective: the psychological impact of not only having a visible difference but of coming into contact with the service as a patient, whether as a child or an adult, and the impact of this on the family. All patients and their families will bring their own agendas to the clinic, dependent on the manner in which they acquired their disfigurement, their age, their own and their family's general coping mechanisms, their hopes and fears, and the information they have gathered beforehand from both the general public and from other professionals. By whatever route they come, their perspectives are likely to be different from those of the professionals, whose views will be both at an individual level and as part of a multidisciplinary team. How well patients' needs are recognized, understood and responded to will depend on the sensitivity and flexibility of the hospital service.

Entry into the system

The way patients normally come into contact with the service will depend on the way in which they acquired their disfigurement. Simply, these can be divided into:

- Congenital: children who are born with visible disfigurements, such as a cleft lip, a syndrome such as Apert's, or a smaller skin blemish, such as a mole.

- Trauma: children or adults who have received severe burns, or disfigurements through an accident, such as a depressed skull fracture, amputation, or facial scarring. The degree to which they were responsible for their disfigurement may affect their attitude to asking for help. In addition, there may be other implications such as litigation for personal injury.
- Evolving: children or adults who develop normally for a time and then gradually develop a disfigurement, such as neurofibromatosis or a rodent ulcer.
- Disease Process: children or adults who have a severe skin complaint that is either intermittent, such as eczema or psoriasis, or permanent, such as scarring from acne or disfigurement following surgery for cancer.

The acquisition of the disfigurement whether from birth, from trauma or from a slow realization, may have a fundamentally different impact on patients and their families, which will affect how they view their approach to the service, how they come into contact with it and what their needs may be.

Evolution of a service

Health care for those with disfigurement has been a slowly evolving service that varies between and within regions. While all regions are likely to have specialist dermatology and plastic surgery clinics, burns units and craniofacial services tend to be supraregional. Often, services are built up on an ad hoc basis, with a consultant developing a specialist interest and gradually creating a team of different professionals over a period of time. In other cases there may be a definite policy decision, followed by the promise of, or bid for, funding. A strategy for delivering a clinical service can then be developed as an integrated whole. The personnel who are initially involved in decision making and planning will define the focus and the way the service is delivered. Thus, the emphasis of a team dominated by the views of the surgeon working within the framework of a medical model will differ in the service it offers compared with one where the work of the staff is driven by a psychological model.

Consequently, clinics and services round the country have a different mix of personnel, despite appearing alike superficially. The importance of stressing this here is that current practice in service delivery differs around the country, at least in the manner in which patients are helped, if not in the overall aim of treatment.

Where there is central government funding for a service, referrals may come from anywhere in the UK, but, if the service is regional, extra-contractual referrals will be necessary, and local referrers may have differing priorities with regard to allocating resources for specialist services.

The emphasis in this section is on the psychological impact of the service on people who are visibly different and, consequently, on the interventions needed. Unfortunately, although health care managers are increasingly aware of the importance of psychological medicine, a psychological service may be delivered only at the patient level, with little opportunity to work at both the systems or strategic planning levels. Yet, the very nature of patients' entry into the health service impinges on many different psychological, as well as medical, issues.

Working practice

What are the psychological needs of such families, and how are they served by the hospital system designed for their care? To what extent can a system heighten the anxiety and distress it purports to reduce, and what implications does this carry for the professionals involved? We shall examine these issues using practices of three types of centre in the UK as examples.

Centre 1: craniofacial clinic for children

New referrals from GPs or, more usually, consultant paediatricians, are initially seen by a consultant neurosurgeon or a plastic surgeon. Diagnoses range from single-suture craniosynostosis to complicated syndromes involving multisuture synostosis (e.g. Crouzon's or Apert's Syndromes).

Children are seen in early infancy, generally within the first few weeks of life. Following this initial appointment, at which the parents would be offered a provisional diagnosis, children are admitted for a four to five-day inpatient assessment, during which time they will undergo a variety of medical tests including: computed tomography (CT) scans, photographs, developmental assessment, genetic opinion, speech therapy opinion, orthoptical, ophthalmological and audiological assessments, social work assessment as appropriate, an interview with a psychologist, and further plastic and neurosurgical assessment.

On the basis of CT scan results, some children will proceed to having their intracranial pressure (ICP) monitored, which will involve a general anaesthetic and a further 24-hour stay in hospital. Parents are given information on whom they will be seeing and a rough timetable, although in practice this is often changed. The child will then go home, usually before all the test results are available and collated.

The consultant neurosurgeon and the plastic surgeon meet with the unit co-ordinator and members of other disciplines at the beginning of the following week to plan treatment. Parents are then informed by letter or telephone and invited for a second outpatient appointment for further discussions about surgery with the consultant whom they originally saw. Depending on the outcome, children are then put on the waiting list for surgery or a list for outpatient follow-up. If the ICP is raised, or urgent surgery is indicated, the child is admitted quickly. Following surgery, the child will be seen regularly for follow-up at outpatient appointments.

Those children requiring further complicated surgery involving functional issues, such as breathing difficulties, are included in monthly craniofacial clinics. These clinics are organized in two parts, consisting of separate morning and afternoon sessions.

In the morning session, the child and family are seen routinely by the clinical psychologist, speech therapist and orthoptist, and may also undergo hearing tests or radiography if necessary. The psychologist uses this meeting to meet the family, if not already known to him or her, to learn the history, and to discuss current concerns and the questions that the family wish to be answered by the surgeons. This assessment will also pick up longer-term issues, for example, bullying at school or a need for specialist help, which may need further liaison with local education authorities or schools. Such interviews can last up to 30 minutes, although in practice families and psychologists often need longer time together.

In the afternoon, patients are seen by the full team simultaneously gathered together in a large room or a hospital lecture theatre. There can be up to 20 people, including junior doctors, nurses and other visitors. Before each family is seen, there is a brief discussion to look at pictures and scans, and to discuss medical issues. The psychologist gives a summary of what has been learned during the morning that is relevant to the appointment. There follows a brief discussion with the patient and family at which future plans are outlined.

Centre 2: a plastic surgery outpatient clinic

Referrals to plastic surgery clinics come from as diverse a range of routes as any other medical discipline. Adults and children may be referred by primary practitioners for congenital, developmental, traumatic and oncological reasons. Secondary and tertiary referrals are very common for complex types of disfigurement and advanced conditions. Plastic surgical opinions are also frequently sought for uncommon conditions, or for 'troubleshooting' complications of conditions usually treated by another discipline. Thus, complex exposed fractures, injuries likely to lead to a disproportionate amount of deformity, or postoperative complications might all find their way into a common general plastic surgery clinic.

Many patients with specific conditions will be directed into specialist joint clinics from the onset. Thus, children with cleft lip and palate will be seen in multidisciplinary clinics involving speech therapists, orthodontists, link nurses, paediatricians, ENT and oral surgeons, photographers, and, hopefully (although by no means always), psychologists. Patients with cancer will be reviewed in combined clinics with representatives of several disciplines present. Patients with potentially embarrassing special needs, such as boys with hypospadias, will usually be seen with an appropriate degree of privacy by a surgeon of the same gender.

A plastic surgery outpatient clinic is generally very busy, with many patients to be seen. Waiting times can be long, whilst the time with the surgeon may be brief. In addition, the consulting room is often a bustling place, with other staff such as nurses and junior doctors observing the consultation. Thus, there may be little opportunity to have a detailed consultation in privacy. This is of particular relevance when the decision about whether to opt for surgery (which is the usual reason for referral in the first place) is a complex one and when the condition to be corrected is not of a life-threatening or physically painful nature. Time should be allowed to discuss possible complications, together with an estimate of the likelihood of a successful outcome for the procedure. If the surgeon becomes uneasy at a perceived mismatch in the patient's expectations of surgery and reality, further consultation is advised. The relatively rare cases of body dysmorphic disorders are referred to a liaison psychiatrist for consideration before any surgical intervention is even broached as a subject.

Once surgery has been planned and fully discussed with the patient (involving children at whatever level is deemed appropriate), the patient is photographed with consent (which is almost universally given and understood by patients). For certain conditions, nursing staff have been trained as link counsellors to reinforce information given during the medical consultation. Such conditions might be breast surgery (reconstructive and aesthetic procedures), skin cancer, head and neck cancer, and deforming skin conditions. Any patient with significant psychosocial or sexual problems relating to the condition and/or subsequent surgery will be referred to the clinical psychologist for advice and management.

Centre 3: neurosurgical intensive care unit

When an adult or child is admitted to intensive care after trauma, perhaps following a road traffic accident resulting in a head injury and/or multiple injuries that are life-threatening, any visible scarring that may have resulted from the accident or come about because of the procedures – for instance, surgery to the face to repair fractures – will be seen, at least initially, as of secondary importance when compared with life-saving procedures. Even as the patient makes a slow recovery, it is possible that visible scarring will not be seen as a major problem compared with functional problems, such as difficulties in walking or speaking, or the more subtle effects on cognitive functioning following a head injury.

If the consequences of the accident have been serious, it may be some months or even years after the accident before a referral is made for craniofacial or plastic surgery. Referrals may come from GPs, a consultant in neurosurgery, or from any field of medicine in which a consultant took the lead in co-ordinating aftercare. While in some cases a referral may be initiated by medical staff, it is equally possible that it is the patient or the family who ask for a referral. If there has been good rehabilitation, then children or adults will already have had the opportunity to discuss their feelings about their changed appearance prior to the referral and arrival at the clinic.

A patient is likely to be seen by the consultant plastic or craniofacial surgeon who will then request various medical investigations including radiographs, photographs, and the opinion of other consultants who may be involved. If the person has not already seen a psychologist, a referral may be crucial, not least in that there may be some specific cognitive impairments, that are not immediately apparent, such as memory loss, or a failure to think through the short- and long-term consequences of a request for surgery. Once medical and psychological opinions have been given, then the patient will be informed of the final decision and eventually admitted for surgery.

Centre 4: the private sector

Self-referral, effectively prevented in the NHS by convention, and, more recently, by funding constraints, is a very common route into private medical consultation. This route is especially valuable for the embarrassed, self-conscious patient, as well as the parent who feel they are seen as over-concerned about their child's problem. In this latter case, the greater time and privacy afforded by the feeling of having 'purchased' the right to medical advice is much valued. In addition, those who practice in the private sector have reached the level of consultants in the NHS, and so the patient knows that he or she will be seen by someone who is fully trained and that there will be continuity of care by the same practitioner. The patient seeking private care also has choice over which practitioner to consult. However, the financial costs can be high and not all treatment is covered by private insurance. This is particularly true of any treatment that is deemed to be 'cosmetic' by the insurers. Patients who are considering private treatment should always establish what the costs are likely to be and how they can be met.

Although the impetus generally comes from the individual, the practitioner will generally require a letter of referral from the patient's own family doctor, who can advise on the most appropriate specialist. This ensures that care is co-ordinated and that relevant medical information is communicated. Once this initial letter of referral is obtained, then the patient can contact the private hospital or clinic and make the first appointment.

There is a word of caution to add here. With the growth and popularity of cosmetic surgery, numerous private clinics have developed, which advertise in the press and in magazines. They often make claims such as being able to make people beautiful and to change their lives. They do not require referral letters from family doctors and may offer credit for easy payment. Once an initial contact has been made, they can then be very persistent in following up that contact. Consultant physicians and surgeons do not generally practice from such clinics, and, although the practitioners may be competent, there are no guarantees that they are trained specialists in their fields. Patients who are in doubt should always consult their family doctor for advice.

Services continue to evolve. This means that in all the four types of service described above, there have been and continue to be changes in service delivery.

Psychological impact of service delivery

The goldfish bowl

One of the problems that those who are visibly different have to overcome is the reaction from the public to their disfigurements, being looked at and responded to as different. This is amply discussed elsewhere in this book, but, as already described above, specialist clinics comprise a large team of professionals who want and/or may need to look at the person in question. For many, especially the children, the feared public gaze is mirrored by the institutional gaze, and is experienced as embarrassing and even hostile. Does the clinic become a circus? Families can feel gaped at so easily.

Communication issues

The goldfish bowl effect can heighten existing anxiety and can have a direct effect on how patients ask questions and process the information. Questions can easily be forgotten, and the professional opinion misheard, misunderstood or not heard. This can cause embarrassment and distress when the patient returns home and the family asks about outcome.

The advantage of seeing many professionals involved in the patient's care can be outweighed by the cumulative effect of large numbers. Many patients will want a clear, definitive solution, and are sometimes confused by the necessary discussions between the various professionals, which go on in front of them. For instance, the neurosurgeon may ask the plastic surgeon for an opinion. Each professional may have a different communication style, so the resultant opinion may be perceived erroneously as discrepant, or even as a disagreement. Patients can go home without a written summary of the consultation: a document which can be helpful to families in understanding the information on which they may have to make major decisions.

Time and distance

There can be a big emotional build-up to hospital attendance, especially if patients are coming for important decisions about surgery. Many have to travel long distances – often well over 150 miles – to attend a clinic, sometimes necessitating an overnight stay. Some hospitals will offer hospital accommodation to children and their parents, but others may not have this facility. Many professionals will need to be involved in the initial assessment and, if patients live a great distance from the hospital, ideally, they do not wish to make multiple journeys that will interrupt school or work and can lead to considerable financial cost. A properly integrated assessment may mean appointments with a surgeon, a radiologist, an ophthalmologist, a psychologist and a speech therapist, as well as members of other departments, which can leave adults, let alone children, extremely tired by the end of the day. This can also be counterproductive to creating a sense of psychological well-being, which is crucial in establishing optimal decision making and treatment outcome. The appointment with the consultant, invariably seen as the most crucial, is often the briefest, which can be very distressing, as patients often want to hear detailed descriptions of the surgery they or their child will undergo, as well as to discuss causation.

Facing up to diagnosis

Anxiety which has been subdued by a previous opinion that 'there is nothing wrong', can now be heightened by hospital attendance. Families will also see other patients with similar problems, possibly at later stages in treatment. While it can be supportive to see others with the same disfigurement, seeing how they look further on in the process can be disillusioning and distressing.

There are a number of issues that patients and their families bring to the clinic: those they want to talk openly about, or explicit issues, and others beneath the surface, or implicit issues:

Explicit issues

Families may ask the following questions:

Why?

Even when there is no known cause for the congenital deformity, parents are anxious to know why it happened *to them*. There is an overriding need to know why, even when there is no known causation (Middleton, 1993). For instance, mothers frequently cite a fall during pregnancy or having always slept in the same position as possible reasons, even when they know this is not the case. If these issues are not openly discussed, even in terms of the impossibility of knowing why, then parents may reach their own erroneous and idiosyncratic reasons, which could affect their relationship with the child and may influence their decision to have other children.

What?

The most important question is: How will it look afterwards? People (adults, parents and their children) need realistic expectations about the final results of surgery. Patients often focus on one particular feature they wish to be changed (e.g. nose shape), not realizing that many procedures may be necessary to correct the underlying facial bone structure. There is also a need for detailed explanations about the procedures themselves (e.g. the short-term effects of surgery, such as pain, discomfort and bruising, and long-term aftercare).

When?

Timing and urgency for cosmetic surgery may differ between adults and children. Adults usually come along after considerable forethought, wanting surgery as soon as possible. On the other hand, some parents of very young children may only be looking to the possibility of surgery in the future. Many parents, naturally, would like all surgery completed by the time their child is due to start school or at least enter secondary school. However, sometimes there are optimal times for certain surgical procedures (e.g. when facial bone growth is completed), which may mean that children have to wait until their teens. Both children and parents may be disappointed that a wait is recommended.

Implicit issues

There may be underlying issues that can profoundly affect the family's interaction with the service.

Failure to accept

This can present in several ways. In infants with craniofacial problems, parents are often shocked by the birth of a child who is perhaps considerably less attractive than most babies. Parents may experience difficulty in bonding with their babies, and, in rare cases, there may be unexpressed recriminations as to whose fault it is. There can be subtle effects upon parent–child interaction, for example, reduced smiling, eye contact and play (Field and Vegha-Lahr, 1984), which may be picked up at the outpatient appointment or during an inpatient assessment.

In older children, who may already have had surgical treatment, there may be subtle messages that parents find the appearance of their children unacceptable, for example, mothers who always clothe their daughters in elaborately pretty dresses to emphasize their femininity. Repeated requests from parents for yet another small operation to straighten the nose, reduce or enhance the cheek or forehead etc. should also be considered as possible indications that parents have not accepted their child for what he or she is.

Clearly, it is important that these issues are carefully and sensitively explored before any treatment or surgery is carried out. If not, the psychological problems are likely to continue and there will be dissatisfaction with treatment.

Anxiety and distress

The psychological distress and anxiety created by visible disfigurement can be quite overt. However, there may also be unresolved issues relating to the shock of the birth (in the case of a child), self-image and lack of confidence, family and public reaction, and hospital experiences that interfere with the patient's ability to express personal wishes coherently and assertively.

The clinic setting itself can engender the very anxiety it seeks to dissipate. Many people do not know what to expect, perhaps because of inadequate preparation by referrers and their own embarrassment. Coming to a hospital, they may feel that, as patients for cosmetic surgery, they may have lower status than those with medical priorities. For many patients, just meeting with a specialist consultant and the associated team may be a daunting experience, irrespective of the sensitive way in which that service is delivered.

This anxiety shows itself in patients who appear to have few questions or who return repeatedly with the same questions. Information may be poorly understood or forgotten, which, in turn, feeds into the spiral of anxiety. Difficulties in remembering can cause embarrassment when returning home to the family who may ask about the outcome.

Fears

As with all hospital admissions, there are often generalized and pervasive fears surrounding anaesthesia, pain and death, which can be unexpressed and therefore underestimated by staff.

Gender issues

Pressure for surgery may be influenced by gender. Parents frequently express greater concern about the future attractiveness of a daughter than of a son with a similar disfigurement. For instance, there may be comments like: 'It wouldn't matter so much for a boy.' More women than men present as patients requesting cosmetic surgery. Initially, fathers may deny the effect of the disfigurement on facial appearance and hence regard surgery as unnecessary, unlike mothers, who may be much more likely to want something done.

Anger

Anger is a very common reaction to visible disfigurement: 'Why me? or, 'Why my child?' This can compound, but should not be confused with the anger generated by the medical system itself. Some patients may have waited a long time for a specialist referral, maybe only discovering by chance that help is available (e.g. a locum GP who happens to know of a specialist team). Many mothers of newborn infants are told that their baby's misshapen head is a result of moulding and are labelled overanxious and neurotic.

Consent

An adult patient requesting surgery is implicitly giving his or her consent. For children, this has to be done on their behalf. Depending on their age and stage of development, their concerns and worries may well differ from those of their parents. Their understanding of the issues, both in the short and long term, will vary, and their agenda may be quite different from that of their parents. As Alderson (1993) has shown, even quite young children can articulate their views and wishes about treatment and surgery, which need to be taken into consideration before any final decisions are made. Therefore, it will be important for parents and the medical team to clarify who wants what and why. This will be discussed further in Chapter 23.

Psychological and social factors that may influence service provision

Although the prime aim of coming to the clinic will be to see if surgical intervention is possible and appropriate, patients and their families will bring other concerns, not necessarily directly relating to their wish for surgery. These concerns can relate to family functioning, difficulties with work or friendships, or to other interpersonal problems. In some instances, these may have been subsumed by the overriding worries about possible surgery and may have been temporarily put aside. They may also occasionally be a major reason for asking for surgery when other management or treatment may be more appropriate. Exploration of this is important not only in helping the team to decide whether surgical intervention is appropriate but also to complement the service offered and to ensure that recovery from surgery can occur in a psychologically supportive environment.

Concerns may relate to:

Family functioning

It is sometimes possible that the birth of a disfigured baby will have affected one or both of the parents' ability to form a strong attachment to the child. Very rarely, this leads to overt rejection. It is more likely that the child will be cared for physically but one parent may find it difficult to love and nurture him or her. This can lead to disagreements in families where one parent is overprotective and the other more distant. Such tensions can be exacerbated if there are feelings of guilt and blame associated with the origin of the disfigurement.

Brothers and sisters of these children may also present with a variety of school, behavioural and emotional problems, which go beyond those arising from normal sibling rivalry. A disfigured child, particularly with a developmental delay, may become so much the focus of parents' attention that there is little time for the needs of other children in the family. Family life becomes centred around the disfigured child. A brother or sister may feel angry (and consequently guilty for feeling angry) towards the unfortunate sibling and the parents, or become so involved with the sibling's care that normal childhood activities are reduced. Friends may feel less happy in visiting the house, and siblings may find themselves bearing the brunt of questioning and perhaps teasing in the playground. Siblings' reactions may be reflected in poor school work or acting out behaviour.

In adults, disfigurement may also result in rejection by family members, isolation from family activities, or development of excessive pity and over-protection. An older member of the family who is suddenly severely disfigured may experience open curiosity and at least temporary fear from young children and perhaps even adult members of the family. It may be hard to cope with this.

Development and intellectual functioning

Concurrent with a number of congenital syndromes, and implicit in those who have received severe head and facial injuries, are issues relating to development and intellectual functioning.

In infants, there may be a number of problems relating to eating and drinking (in the case of cleft palate for instance) or breathing and sleeping (in children who have small nasal passages such as in Apert's and Crouzon's syndromes). When a baby is born with hand anomalies, such as fused fingers, fine motor co-ordination will be delayed until surgery has been performed. Gross motor skills and speech can be delayed and, where there is raised intracranial pressure, intellectual functioning can also be affected. In such cases, parents are likely to be concerned not only about how their child looks but also how the child will develop in the future and if they will eventually be able to function independently.

Education and work

There is considerable evidence that people make negative discriminations and attributions about those with visible disfigurement (Bull and Rumsey, 1988). Patients attending clinics are often concerned about the public's reaction to them in the street and the wrong assumptions based solely on their appearance that employers and teachers make about their abilities. Adults may choose a form of work where they have little contact with the general public, and children are given less opportunities in school to show their real abilities.

Friendships and attachments

Not only may school and work experiences and achievements have been affected by a patient's disfigurement but the person's life style may also have resulted in a real or self-imposed isolation. Very young children may not be affected to any great degree, but, as they get older, they are likely to become more aware of their disfigurement and its effect on their ability to make close friends. Living and going to school in a close community may mean that during the primary school years a child is relatively protected and friendships are made, although this is not always the case. Entry into a large comprehensive school and the coming of puberty, however, can enhance the self-consciousness of disfigurement and result in more difficulties in making friends. Adolescents and adults may fear that they will be unable to make close and lasting adult relationships and perhaps isolate themselves from society in order to protect themselves from rejection. Some may become depressed when they consider how their disfigurement may affect their personal and work prospects. The extent to which they feel that surgery would provide the solution to these problems needs to be explored.

Overt hostility

Teasing and bullying are frequent concerns raised by parents and children at clinics. This can occur in the classroom, the playground or in the neighbourhood. Adults, too, can experience bullying at work, as well as encountering intrusive staring or unpleasant remarks in the street.

Short and long-term implications for intervention

Psychosocial care should be an integral part of all nursing situations; depending on the unit, there may also be professionals, such as clinical psychologists, clinical nurse specialists or social workers, to offer patients specific psychological interventions, both in the short and long term. Each discipline will bring its own particular training, theoretical framework and experience. The mix or overlap of skills can be a source of great enrichment to a unit, even at the risk of occasional professional conflict!

Any intervention will include some or all of the following processes:

- Explanation: providing the opportunity to go over surgical details and correct misheard or misinterpreted information;
- Elicitation: of fears and anxieties about immediate surgery, the future in school or the workplace, which may affect decisions to request or refuse surgical intervention;
- Discussion: helping with decision-making processes, preparation for surgery, or debriefing from the outpatient clinic;
- Liaison: with other appropriate services (e.g. school psychological service or speech therapy), schools, colleges, workplace, other families and self-help groups;
- Shuttle diplomacy: acting as 'go-between' for child and parents, patients and surgeons, particularly when there are differing perceptions of need for or urgency of treatment.

The clinical psychologist may be in a particularly good position to offer these services as a more 'neutral' professional who is not directly involved with medical or surgical care. Patients can often be more critical of services or openly express dissatisfaction over appearance (or the outcome of previous surgery) with a psychologist, rather than the consultant surgeon. The kinds of assessment and treatment that clinical psychologists provide include the following:

Specific psychological assessment and treatment provision

Short-term assessment

- Assessment of developmental and intellectual functioning: an essential part of treatment when diagnosis of visible disfigurement also carries implications for possibly delayed/impaired development;
- Assessment and treatment of behavioural and emotional problems;
- Assessment and treatment of family functioning when there is a problem related to a family member with a visible disfigurement (e.g. problem with acceptance by a sibling or parent);
- Assessment and management of teasing and bullying: teaching specific techniques to cope at school, in public and at work;
- Assertiveness and social skills training, individually or in groups to improve confidence and raise self-esteem.

Long-term assessment

Intervention must be aimed at continually improving services and the effectiveness of treatment offered. This can be done through:

- Audit: development of outcome measures of client, referrer and surgical satisfaction, and examination of any mismatch between these;
- Clinical research:
    To provide long-term psychological and developmental outcome data;
    To develop and test new treatment methods;
- Public relations: to raise public awareness and tolerance of visible disfigurement (e.g. by providing teaching and training in schools and the workplace);

- Training: for other professionals in the field;
- Policy development: strategic planning and development of appropriate services for those with disfigurements.

Conclusion

In summary, coming into contact with different types of service can raise many issues, some of which may not immediately be apparent. The service itself may unwittingly mirror the very difficulties the patient faces in everyday life. The challenge for professional providers is to deliver a flexible and sensitive service, which allows the patient to gain the information they need and the chance to openly express their thoughts and feelings.

References

Alderson, P. (1993). *Children's Consent to Surgery*. Buckingham: Open University Press.

Bull, R. and Rumsey, N. (1988). *The Social Psychology of Facial Appearance*. New York: Springer Verlag.

Field, T.M. and Vegha-Lahr, N. (1984). Early interactions between infants with craniofacial anomalies and their mothers. *Infant Behav. Dev.*, 7, 527–530.

Middleton, J. (1993). *Clinical Audit: Cranio-facial Outpatient Department*. Oxford: The Radcliffe Infirmary.

Chapter 23

Patient involvement in decision making about treatment

Eileen Bradbury with Judith Middleton

Those with a visible difference often have considerable contact with surgical and other medical professionals, who may offer physical treatment to improve appearance and/or function. Making decisions about whether or not to have treatment can be difficult for individuals and their families. This chapter addresses the issue of decision making about physical treatment and how that process can be facilitated in order to ensure that individuals and their families are able to be involved in decisions that affect them.

The decision-making process

When people make decisions, they usually weigh up the costs and benefits: 'What will I get out of this and what will I have to do to get it?' They are affected by factors such as availability: 'How easy is it to get the outcome?', confirmation of expectations: 'Does it fit with what I expect or want?' and the influence of ethical values: 'Is it what I ought to do?' There are other factors that influence decision making, such as commitment to the outcome and the influence of other people. Even for relatively straightforward decisions, the process of decision making is often a mixture of beliefs, values and emotional judgements.

The aim of the decison-making process within the context of disfigurement is to arrive at a stable decision that can be sustained and that feels to be the right decision for that person. To make such a decision, there are five main stages (Janis and Mann, 1977):

1. *Appraising the challenge* In order to do this, a person needs to understand what can be achieved and what the cost will be in terms of hospitalization, pain, potential complications and inconvenience (short-term costs), and secondary scarring and potential long-term complications (long-term costs). Part of the process of appraising the challenge requires an understanding of what personal and social resources a person possesses to meet this challenge and what they need.

2. *Surveying alternatives* There is often more than one way of treating a physical problem. For someone with a birthmark to the face, alternatives can include laser treatment, tissue expansion or cosmetic camouflage. In order to survey alternatives, the person needs to have comprehensive and comprehensible information. This may involve talking to other doctors in other specialties and can be a laborious business. People may feel that they have to accept what has been offered and that they are not being a 'good patient' if they ask for another opinion or try something else.
3. *Weighing alternatives* This can be difficult. Once more, good information is the key, but the person may need particular help in weighing up the costs and benefits of each alternative. It is at this stage that they are most likely to be influenced by prior beliefs and commitments and by their emotional state.
4. *Reaching commitment* This stage can come as a great relief, as it is a resolution of all that has gone before. The person may have spent much time agonizing over the decision. In order to proceed with the decision, there needs to be a process of commitment to the chosen course of action. During this process, additional evidence in support of the decision is focused upon, and evidence that weighs against the decision is given less priority or discarded.
5. *Adherence to the decision* Once the decision is firmly made, the person needs to be able to adhere to that decision. It is important that the individual is encouraged to recognize that he or she has made the best decision possible and, whatever its outcome, it was not wrong; the best decision possible was made at that time.

The decision-making process for those with a visible difference

Decision making for those with a visible difference can be fraught with difficulties. Most people go to health care professionals because they are ill or need advice over health issues. For some patients with a visible disfigurement, vital functions are compromised (e.g. breathing and feeding in children with cleft lip and palate, and in some craniofacial syndromes). Those badly scarred by burns may benefit from surgery in terms of a reduction in skin contractures that are causing deformity and loss of function. However, many people with a visible disfigurement form a distinct group in that their primary concerns may not be directly 'medical', but are focused on appearance, which may cause the psychological and social problems described elsewhere in this book. This means that requests for treatment are underpinned by many complex psychological issues that are not directly related to physical health. These issues may not be immediately apparent and their exploration is a crucial prerequisite to surgical planning.

Relief may be experienced when there are also medical reasons for surgery (e.g. signs of raised intracranial pressure). Conversely, if there is no medical urgency, anxiety may be raised as prospective patients weigh up the subjective and hoped-for improvement in appearance against the risks of surgery and the stress of a hospital admission. They may also be concerned that others will disapprove of treatment for a cosmetic, nonmedical problem.

There are problems inherent in the decision-making process for those with a visible difference. These include:

- *Popular beliefs about the 'magic' of plastic surgery* This can lead to a futile search for the complete cure. The search can be driven by friends and relatives who may induce feelings of guilt in the parents of or the person with the disfigurement; they may suggest that the 'cure' is available and the person has failed to make the effort to find it.
- *The numbers of professionals involved in the treatment* There may be several professionals involved in the treatment, for example, children with cleft lip and palate can see surgeons, orthodontists, speech and language therapists, ENT specialists, psychologists etc. If the treatment is not co-ordinated, decisions about one aspect can interfere with decisions about others. There is also the problem of communicating needs and gaining information from many different people, and there may be many hospital visits; not every member of the family who wants to be involved in making decisions can keep up with all these visits.
- *Lack of certainty of outcome* Some of the treatments on offer may be experimental, and few will guarantee results. This makes it difficult to decide what to do.

Facilitating the decision-making process

People struggling to make decisions about treatment can be helped with this process, which can be facilitated in the following ways:

Clarifying the aims and objectives

Although there may be common psychological and social problems experienced by those with disfigurement, these are mediated by individual differences. People will have particular aims and objectives as they consider surgery, but these may not be clear to those involved or to the professionals treating them. It is difficult to make decisions when the individual's personal circumstances are not known.

For example, surgery can be carried out to transfer the great toe from the foot to the hand following a hand injury where the thumb is lost. This leaves the foot with a clear deficit, and the hand with a strong new 'thumb'. For the working man who needs his hands for his employment, the transfer makes sense. For the man whose main hobby is amateur athletics, then the loss of the toe would be a problem and the decision is less clear.

The more complex the decision, the more care should be taken to clarify aims.

Providing information

As described above, people need relevant and accessible information in order to make decisions; this may be written or verbal. Written information can be in the form of preprinted information sheets, articles or books. It can also be prepared especially for those who attend a particular clinic with a defined problem. Verbal information is very variable in its usefulness. There is a tendency for clinicians to use their own language without even realizing that others may not understand; thus 'sutures' may be used instead of 'stitches', 'GA' instead of 'general anaesthetic' or 'being put to sleep', and 'melanoma' instead of 'skin cancer'. Even seemingly nonmedical words can baffle and confuse. For example, one study showed that only 48% of the population understand the word 'fatal' and 70% the meaning of 'harmful' (Ley *et al.*, 1985).

In order to ensure that the person is fully informed of the situation and that this information has been conveyed accurately, it is important for the clinician to think about the language used, to say things in different ways and to check out that it has been understood. For the individual involved, it is important that they should feel able to ask when they do not understand, to pose questions if they wish to expand their knowledge, and to ensure that the information they are given is relevant to their needs. Bringing prepared written questions can help. The clinician should encourage this as it is likely to lead to better quality interaction.

Contact with former patients

Sometimes people need to gather information from others who have been through the same treatment or have the same condition. It is useful to keep a list of people who are willing to be contacted for such purposes. In addition, support groups can put people in touch with each other. There should be a list of such support groups with contact numbers in every clinic where treatment decisions are being discussed. For a discussion of the advantages and disadvantages of support groups see Chapter 27.

Assessing and working with underlying issues

As well as receiving information, the person and/or the family may need time to work through other issues that can cloud the decision-making process. Parents who are still actively upset about their baby's disfigurement will find it difficult to make a decision, and need time to express their thoughts and feelings in a therapeutic environment. Adults who have unexpressed distress may become tearful in clinic when treatment is discussed. They, too, would benefit from taking time to talk this through before making any decision about treatment.

Supportive counselling that promotes discussion in an empathic and accepting way will help to ensure the treatment decisions are made in the best interests of the person involved (Bradbury *et al.*, 1994a).

Giving the child a voice: the competence of children to make decisions

The issue of children's competence to be involved in the decision-making process is an important one. Parents and doctors are often faced with the issue of surgery and other forms of treatment for children that may not change their physical functioning but which alters their appearance.

Parents may say, 'What will she say when she is 14? How can I make a decision for her? At what age can she make that decision herself?'

There is a legal requirement for parents of children under the age of 16 years to sign the consent form for treatment, but, in practice, children have an increasing say in their treatment as they get older, and few doctors would override the wishes of an adolescent. In the Gillick case (1985), Lord Scarman ruled that a child under 16 years, who showed 'a sufficient understanding and intelligence to understand fully what is proposed', was competent to give or to withhold consent to treatment. However, despite legal debate, the issue of children's consent to treatment remains unclear and, in practice, the extent of a child's involvement is frequently left to the judgement of the clinician and parents.

However, both these groups of adults may be driven by their own needs. The clinicians may feel committed to a type of treatment, or may hold strong beliefs about whether children should have treatment. The problems some parents have in adjusting to the birth of a baby with a visible disfigurement, and the guilt parents often feel when a child has a disfiguring injury, have been described elsewhere in this book. Decision making for children can be fraught with problems relating to the parents' own needs to resolve their feelings, and, in such cases, decisions to undergo surgery may be of greater benefit to the parent than the child (Bradbury *et al.*, 1994b). Alderson (1993) has shown that young children can make stable and reasonable decisions and could make informed choices if adults had communicated the issues to them in language they could understand. However, other writers have shown that even adolescents can be manipulated in a clinic when discussing treatment by directed questioning and selective listening.

The importance of relevant and comprehensible information for adults has already been discussed. It is particularly important for children, who may find it difficult to understand all the nuances of adult conversation. In addition, some thought needs to be given to the environment in which this information is conveyed and discussed.

Creating a clinic environment in which effective decisions can be made

Both adults and children may find that the environment of the outpatient clinic – where most medical decisions are made – is a difficult one in which to communicate effectively. There are many reasons for this. The average surgical outpatient clinic is very busy. Each appointment may only last a few minutes because of the sheer pressure of numbers. In addition, the room may be noisy and bustling with people coming and going. It is very difficult to give and receive information in this environment. If the physical environment of such a clinic cannot be changed, then those facing complex treatment decisions should be given a separate appointment with a professional such as a liaison nurse, who can help the person reach a decision. This may be appropriate at the time, in a separate room, or on a different day. Even within the confines of such a clinic, the medical professional should ensure that the information given is understood, and that information is gathered about the aims and objectives of the prospective patient.

People with congenital conditions, such as cleft lip and palate, may attend multidisciplinary clinics. The potential problems associated with such clinics have been described in Chapter 22. They may provide a hostile environment for young people: there can be many unknown adults who control the conversation; the child may feel too much the centre of adult attention; and the physical environment may be bleak, with tangible reminders of treatment, such as trays of instruments. When there are decisions to be made about treatment, it is generally appropriate to take the child, with or without the family, to a separate quiet room where the issues can be discussed. The younger child should be seen with the family and given toys to play with to reduce the tension, and also have drawing facilities available to help communication. The adolescent is often best seen alone, to give him or her a chance to talk things through in private and without professional or family intrusion.

Empowering patients to say 'no' to treatment

Just as people need to feel empowered to be involved in the process of making decisions about having treatment, they also need to be able to say 'no' to treatment, or 'no more' to further treatment. This is a very difficult process for the individual. It can mean:

- They are disappointing their family and friends, who may be encouraging the treatment process;
- They are disappointing the clinician, who has been so good to them and who may seem keen on the treatment;
- They are letting go of hopes for further improvement and now have to come to terms with how they look.

It can be much harder to refuse treatment than to accept it. There are many reasons why a person may want to say no:

- They may not want to face going through the treatment again.
- They may feel that it is important to come to terms with how they look and need the opportunity to do that.
- They may feel that they have been lucky so far and not want to risk anything going wrong.

Whatever the reasons, these need to be acknowledged and respected. The drive for treatment can overwhelm a person's individual needs. It may require someone other than the clinician who is treating the individual to listen away from the clinic and to empower that person to speak out and say what they do and do not want.

Decision making after head injury (Judith Middleton)

Accidents that cause facial disfigurement may be associated with head injury. Even after a relatively mild head injury, a person may have some disturbance of thinking and decision making, although this is likely to be of a temporary nature. After more serious head injuries, however, previous intellectual abilities may be subtly, but importantly, changed for a long time if not permanently. Particular problems may include evaluating information, predicting future events in a reasonable manner and making rational decisions. In addition, some people with head injuries become less flexible in how they try to solve problems and, despite contradictory evidence, will continue to pursue a certain solution very persistently. They may also be obsessed with pursuing their goal, despite reasonable advice to the contrary, and be less sensitive to other people's opinions and feelings.

These sometimes subtle changes in personality and thinking can mean that friends and close relatives find the person becomes quite different, and, after a time, may react differently, perhaps in some cases becoming less friendly. Thus, there can be a loss of old friends and an equally greater difficulty in making new friends after a head injury.

If the person also has some visible difference that has resulted from the injury, this may be blamed for the change in social relationships, although, in effect, it is the subtle personality changes that are at the root of the problem. This means that patients may request plastic surgery in order to change their appearance in the mistaken belief that this will redress their social isolation and their other difficulties. Any suggestion that surgery may not bring about the changes they want will be dismissed, and they persistently make the same request to the same plastic surgeon or may shop around until they find a surgeon who will operate.

Prior to any plastic surgery for cosmetic reasons for a person who has suffered a head injury, a careful assessment should be made of the individual's ability to make an informed and reasonable decision. This should be based on the present level of cognitive functioning rather than that prior to the injury. Counselling and advice should be offered, but a longer than usual time may be needed to reach an appropriate decision. Conversely, and very occasionally, those with insight into their cognitive difficulties may want to keep some disfigurement as a visible sign or 'badge' to give others some indication of their difficulties.

Conclusions

Thus, there are factors within decision making that do need to be addressed for people with a visible difference. Physical treatment carries with it so many hopes and aspirations, and yet also has so many uncertainties. Motivation for treatment may be profoundly affected by unresolved emotional issues. The needs of the individual should be understood and responded to, whether or not the decision is to have treatment. Professionals who treat those with a visible difference should be aware of these issues. There may be a need for additional psychological help in order to facilitate the decision-making process.

References

Alderson, P. (1993). *Children's Consent to Surgery*. Buckingham: Open University Press.
Bradbury, E.T., Kay, S.P.J. and Hewison, J. (1994a). The psychological impact of microvascular free toe transfer for children and their parents. *J. Hand Surg. [Br.]*, **19B**, 689–695.
Bradbury, E.T., Kay, S.P.J., Tighe, C.T. and Hewison, J. (1994b) Decision-making by parents and children in paediatric hand surgery. *Br. J. Plast. Surg.*, **47**, 324–330.

Gillick v. West Norfolk and Wisbech AHA [1985] ER 423.
Janis, I.L. and Mann, L. (1977). *Decision Making: A Psychological Analysis of Conflict, Choice and Commitment*. New York: Free Press.
Ley, P. (1988). *Communicating with Patients*. London: Croom Helm.

Chapter 24

Understanding the problems

Eileen Bradbury

In the first section of this book, individuals have given their own accounts of their experiences, their emotional responses and the reactions of people close to them. Themes that recur in these accounts have been extracted in order to look at problems that can arise, to look at coping techniques that can lead to further problems, and to suggest ways in which individuals can be helped to cope more effectively.

The effect on the individual

Problems that can arise

Many of the writers described their own emotional responses to their visible difference. Three particular themes emerged:

Feelings of being different

'The cruellest legacy of my acne is the profound conviction that I'm different to others'... (Jane, page 61).

Although this perception of difference is often reinforced by the responses of others, it is essentially a personal experience. It can cause the individual to feel very isolated and alone. Working with this issue, the person offering support needs to understand and empathize with this feeling. This understanding is based on a knowledge of the experience of disfigurement gained from reading the literature and also on a process of empathetic and effective listening, which allows the helper to relate to the individual in a therapeutic way. Individuals may feel that no-one understands how they feel; building a therapeutic relationship can diminish that sense of difference and aloneness.

Support groups can also help this process, as long as they do not create a small coterie of people who reinforce their sense of difference (see Chapter 27). Belonging to other social networks within society can help: the Scouts, the local Working Men's Club, etc. Understanding and emphasizing the similarities and joint interests that people share within a structured social environment can help them to share a common humanity.

Loss of identity

'The old Kwasi is there, somewhere, at the core, but it is not possible for me to get back to him' (Kwasi, page 59).

Following a traumatic injury, there can be an identity crisis in which the person loses a sense of self. This can include the sense of family and racial identity. The inability to recognize oneself represents a profound disruption of body image and a major life crisis; the responses are often akin to grieving responses to other types of loss. There can be denial, anger, distress, mourning and yearning, anxiety and depression. As with other forms of loss, there is generally a process of adaptation as the person gradually comes to accept the loss. This can take a long time and help may be needed to cope with this process.

Bereavement counselling can be useful. In his book on grief counselling (1991), Worden describes four tasks of mourning:

1. *To accept the reality of the loss* The person with a disfiguring injury may deny the reality of the loss by refusing to look and/or by adopting an unrealistic view of what treatment can achieve. This denial can be a useful coping strategy; it allows the person a breathing space to recover strength and resources. It allows that sense of optimism that can give energy and a sense of self-efficacy. However, if it goes on too long, and if others use it to help them to feel better, then it delays the task of mourning and the process of adaptation.

2. *To work through the pain and grief* This is a holding process, encouraging the person to express emotions by offering a secure and supportive holding relationship. It is often easier for someone not personally involved to do this. The individual who is experiencing a loss of identity realizes that family and friends may also be experiencing a similar grieving response and therefore may be less emotionally available and too vulnerable to help in an effective way. Those people may well need support themselves.

3. *To adjust to the environment in which the deceased (or the physical other) is missing* This task is one of adaptation, to adjust to the physical changes that have happened and the ways in which those changes influence the person's social environment. It will certainly take time and proceed along an uneven course; sometimes it will feel as though the person is back to square one, but, with help and encouragement to find ways of coping with the altered environment, the individual can gradually adapt to the changes that have happened.

4. *To relocate the loss emotionally and to move on with life* For those who have lost part of their physical identity, the last of these tasks is to relocate that loss within oneself, to recognize and integrate the old self with the new. This can be helped by working with photos taken before the accident and identifying what can be recognized of the altered appearance: the eyes, the build, the posture, the tilt of the head, all those things that make the individual unique and recognizable. This is sensitive work, which can only be done once the other tasks of mourning have been undertaken and resolved within a supportive and therapeutic relationship.

In addition to relocating the physical presence, it is important to help people to recognize continuities in terms of personality. They may feel that the physical changes are reflected in changes to them as people. They may also find that their post-traumatic emotional state is such that they do not recognize their own responses and feel that they have lost the person that they were. Encouraging the individual and the family to identify continuities is of value at such times. This process can be helped by understanding some of the post-traumatic responses. They are described in more detail in the case study of Geoff in the next chapter.

Anxiety

'My lack of experience in social skills meant that I still feared people' (Lisa, page 65).

Those with a visible difference may feel that they lack social confidence. The social skills that are required to deal with the responses of others to disfigurement are more extensive than when there is no disfigurement. We have already seen that people often respond to those with disfigurement in ways that can reflect awkwardness, embarrassment or even hostility. As the result of experiencing these reactions, those born with a visible difference may have withdrawn socially, and may not have gained the social confidence needed to handle the reactions of others. Those with acquired disfigurement may have found that old patterns of social behaviour no longer work so well.

Helping someone to develop social skills and thus to gain confidence in social interactions requires an understanding of the problems disfigured people experience and of why others react as they do. Helping an individual to reach this understanding can encourage him or her to gain a sense of efficacy and control in dealings with other people (see Chapter 18). It is also important to appreciate the individual's strengths, such as a supportive family, a good problem-solving ability, a sense of self-efficacy, and a sense of humour. The individual can be helped to become the 'expert' in handling social situations, by treating the problems as familiar and understandable, and by exploring and developing ways of interacting with others.

Effective social interaction with acquaintances and friends requires social skill. It has much to do with feelings of self-confidence and self-worth. Someone who has experienced a disfiguring injury may feel that friends will now behave differently, that they will reject, pity, or even fail to recognize them in the street. This can happen, and may lead the person to avoid familiar activities and social events.

Such an individual can be helped by encouraging understanding of the responses of others, by finding ways of answering awkward questions, and by developing ways of talking to others. The sense of loss of identity described above can make this process difficult. Helping the person to deal with the issues of identity can help that person gain the confidence to re-establish relationships with others.

Ways in which people have tried to cope

Overcompensation

'I came across as overconfident and brash. It's overcompensation. If you are pretty, you forget how much you use that as a form of communication.... Now I have to rely on my personality' (Wheatley, 1993).

Although this can seem like a useful coping mechanism, it can alienate others. In addition, it may rob the individual who seems so confident, of the ability to elicit support when needed. It is so difficult to express neediness when everyone sees you as strong and coping. Developing a sensitive understanding of the effect one has on others is a useful tool in social interaction, and requires one to observe and understand the reactions of others.

Suppression of emotions

'I think now that I had this strange numbness because I'd have been overwhelmed if I had experienced my real feelings. They would have been too unbearable, so I denied them and buried them' (Jane, page 62).

Suppression of emotions and denial can be a useful way of coping in the short term. It gives breathing space and time to build one's strength. However, if it leads to long-term avoidance of true feelings, it can cause problems. The individual may feel isolated from others and not understood. There may be upsurges of anger and feelings of depression. Those close to the person may feel frustrated by that person's refusal to talk and not know what to say.

The individual can be helped by being given the opportunity to talk openly in a warm and supportive therapeutic situation. He or she may feel afraid of being overwhelmed by the emotions if they are admitted, and it is important that the person who is facilitating this process can allow these emotions to be expressed and receive them in a caring and nonjudgemental way. Sometimes it is useful to work with others in the family; the partner may want to share this experience and can then offer appropriate support. Also, those close to the individual who is disfigured may need to express their own feelings and needs. Facilitating communication between family members can be of great benefit in the healing process.

The responses of strangers

Problems that can arise

Invasion of privacy

'They were so intrigued that they rounded up as many of their friends, relatives and anyone else that was interested to join their group and continue staring, pointing and discussing me' (Marc, page 28).

Those with disfigurement have to deal with the reactions of strangers on a daily basis. They often feel that their privacy has been invaded, that they have become highly visible and thus vulnerable to emotional harm. If this becomes a major problem, then they may stay at home, away from others.

It is not possible to prevent people reacting as they do. The reasons for these reactions have been discussed in Section Two. However, it is possible to help the person with disfigurement to reduce the perception of visibility and vulnerability. The person may find that he or she is walking down the street with a heightened vigilance, watching the faces of others in order to see if they are looking. This can be modified by behavioural strategies, such as unfocusing the eye and not seeing others, and by cognitive strategies, such as concentrating on other thoughts or by thinking of others as being unaware of what they are doing and therefore not trying to do harm. The first of these involves avoidance of the threat, the last involves a reappraisal of the threat.

For example, there is the problem of the initial encounter with a stranger. There is often a short 'stand-off' period at such times when the individual can seize the initiative and decide what to do whilst the stranger is struggling with finding what to say or do. Ways of coping include making contact by smiling and introducing oneself, or turning away and moving off in a purposeful way. The most successful strategy is the one that works best for the individual at that time.

Social rejection

'As the bus starts to move a window on the upper deck slides open. A youth puts his mouth to the window and yells, 'Hi ya flat nose' (John, page 31).

Sometimes the threat is obvious and intrusive, and thus difficult to reappraise. Its meaning is clear. In this situation, the person can gain a feeling of control by learning strategies for ignoring. It requires a sort of protective barrier to be erected. One way of doing this can be described as the 'force-field', the person imagines that he or she is protected by an invisible force-field and insults are like arrows. They hit the force-field and are deflected back. This is a form of visualization that some people, particularly children who are being teased, find very useful. When the person does not respond to the taunts, then the victimization often ceases.

Of course there is always the sheer joy of the clever response, which throws the other person off guard; after all, the individual with disfigurement has plenty of time to think up responses, as the insults usually follow a banal and predictable course. It can help to go over the incident afterwards and to role-play what one would like to have said.

Misconceptions

'Mummy, has that lady got chickenpox?' (Jane, page 62).

Such misconceptions can be troubling and upsetting. The individual then has to decide whether to correct the misconception or to ignore it. This very much depends on the situation. A concerned query can be answered in a relaxed way, although a comment in passing is probably best left. Understanding that such misconceptions are based on lack of knowledge rather than maliciousness is important. This is another way in which the threat can be reappraised.

For all these problems to do with reactions of strangers, it may be helpful to rehearse what could be said and to report back on whether a particular strategy has been effective.

Ways in which people have tried to cope

Social withdrawal

'Most of my school years were spent wandering alone around the play-ground' (Katherine, page 22).

In response to the reactions described above, many people with disfigurement keep out of the way. Although this can be protective, it can also be lonely and does limit a person's ability to develop supportive social networks. An important component of resilience, the ability to withstand adversity, is the development of coping strategies for solving problems. Social experience may be problematic for those with a visible difference, but avoiding social situations does not allow such strategies to be developed. People can be helped by social skills work in order to develop effective ways of interacting with others, they can also be helped by talking through their social experiences and modifying their beliefs about other people, for example, by helping someone to understand that others are feeling embarrassed because they do not know what to say can empower that person to take the social initiative and handle the situation more effectively.

As well as encouraging the development of coping strategies, contact with others allows friendships to grow. Parents can help this process by encouraging their child to invite someone home after school and by including potential friends in family outings. Adults may also need to work actively at developing friendships and take the initiative in suggesting joint activities such as going to the cinema. Both children and adults having visible differences may be held back from such initiatives by a fear of rejection. They can be helped with encouragement to make the first move, and with help in dealing with feelings of rejection if the plan does not work out. It is important to help them to identify whether or not the other person has actually rejected them. If so, it is valuable to focus on what could be done differently next time. Coping with failure is an important element of general coping skills.

It is also important to help people to realize that failure may have nothing to do with the disfigurement. It could be the consequence of an unwise choice of companion or a lack of understanding of how to relate to others. This insight helps them to feel more optimistic about their ability to change things in the future.

Responses of the family

Problems that can arise

Avoidance by the family

'I walk away feeling even more lonely and vulnerable. This is the only time that my father refers to my disfigurement' (John, page 32).

Sometimes family members find it very difficult to cope with a child's disfigurement. Parents may worry about upsetting the child by referring to his or her appearance, although it is more likely that such behaviour is the result of the parents' own difficulties in handling their own emotions. In this situation, the parents need help rather than the child. Working with the parents and helping them to talk through their feelings of guilt, responsibility, anger and/or helplessness can be of great benefit to both parties. It is better that the child is helped by parents rather than professionals. Helping the parents to help the child can encourage normal patterns of family support. Part of this work might be to encourage the parents to feel competent to do this. Parents may feel deskilled because they do not know how best to help their child. Building the confidence and competence of the parents can be a most valuable way of helping the family.

When the child has hospital treatment, then professionals do temporarily take over the care. The more the parents can be involved in the decision making about treatment and the care of their child in hospital, the more they will feel that they are playing a competent parenting role.

If the person with a visible difference is an adult in the family, then it may be up to him or her to take the initiative in discussions. Others may feel that they do not know what to say, or worry that they will say the wrong thing. They may also feel ashamed of their own emotions and distress and not feel entitled to these feelings. The person with the visible difference can be helped to understand how others are feeling through joint discussions. In this way, others in the family can learn to offer appropriate and useful support.

Lack of communication

'We as parents were very worried and upset to find out, years later, how much she had been bullied at school and for how long' (Lisa's parents, page 66).

It may be that the child does not find it easy to communicate with the parents. Children are protective of their parents; they do not want to upset them. Thus they may not tell their parents about the problems that they are experiencing. Parents may be worried about their child, they may be sending 'coded' messages that they do not actually want to know.

Facilitating communication within the family is important, as this can help the family members to support each other. Sitting down with them and encouraging them to talk through the issues can help this process. However, in order fully to appreciate the problems, it may initially be helpful to work with the parents and the child separately, before subsequently working with the family as a group.

Ways in which people have tried to cope

Overprotection

'We [Anthony and his mother] are very close, too close perhaps. Not having a family of my own and finding difficulty in forming relationships, I still, at forty-nine years of age, see her as an emotional crutch.... She remains my main confidante' (Anthony, page 51).

It is very easy to understand why parents wish to protect children with visible differences from unnecessary burdens and unhappiness. At times this means that children can become so protected that they fail to have the normal experiences of childhood that prepare them for adult life. While real anxieties and fears need to be accepted, parents need to be encouraged to help their child to independence and autonomy as far as possible. If children have been the special focus of their parents' attention in early life, due to the circumstances of their disfigurement and subsequent treatment, it can be particularly difficult for parents to relinquish their hold. This can be for a number of reasons.

First of all, children with a visible difference may be more vulnerable than other children not only because of their appearance but also because their life experience in terms of hospital treatment may have meant time off school and away from friends and family. In addition, some conditions in which the brain is also involved may give rise to concurrent cognitive problems, which can include a failure to appreciate danger and real difficulties in coping with unforeseen problems, which occur in everyday life. Parents thus see themselves as the natural barrier between a hostile world and their child.

Secondly, normal development involves a growing independence away from parents, who can find this hard to face even when there are no specific problems.

Thirdly, there are occasions when the apparent dependence of the child on the parents masks a real dependence of parents in having their child at home. If parents have spent many years focusing their lives on their child's well-being and treatment, the loss of this focus as he/she becomes more independent can mean that they have difficulties in becoming a 'couple' again. If there is a single parent, the loss may feel even greater.

Disentangling normal childhood and adolescent experiences from an unrealistic desire for independence is a first step in helping families. Encouraging parents to allow children to experience limited dangers so that they can learn coping strategies for themselves is another important step. Parents should also be given the opportunity to explore dependency issues and be offered support in restructuring their lives without the child as the focus. All this needs to be done slowly and with great sensitivity if both the child and the parents are to reach independence from each other and also remain interdependent in an appropriate way.

Experiences at school

Problems that may arise

Teasing and rejection by children at school

'I have come to the conclusion that school was the biggest contributing factor to the way I feel about my face now' (Lisa, page 64).

School is the main social arena of the child. Social isolation and/or rejection makes it difficult for the child to gain the social skills necessary to form satisfactory relationships in adult life. It can reinforce the feelings of difference described above. It can also interfere with learning, as this is often carried out as a group activity.

Children who are visibly different are often the subject of teasing and bullying. Despite being upset by this, they may not tell their parents or teachers. However, they may show reluctance to attend school or go out to play; they may look generally sad or start showing disruptive behaviour. It is therefore always important to ask not only parents but also the children themselves (perhaps in the absence of their parents) if teasing has occurred, how this was dealt with and the effectiveness of any strategies used.

When children do admit to being bullied or teased, this should be taken seriously and immediate inquiries should be made at the school. Schools vary in how they approach the issue of teasing and parents may need to talk not only to the class teacher but also to the head teacher. Even if this is not a current worry, parents are frequently concerned that teasing will occur in the future, especially when children move to other schools. Advice and support about what to do are often sought.

This can be offered by working directly with children to help them to learn how to assert themselves in a nonaggressive way in difficult situations. Various tricks can also be suggested about how they can shield themselves from unkind comments. Some social skills training can be helpful. This work may be carried out in schools or in specialist clinics, or through voluntary organizations such as the charity Changing Faces, which runs workshops for these kinds of problems (see contact address in Chapter 27).

Parents can be instrumental in preventing problems from arising at the transition periods (e.g. school entry, change of school) by approaching the school before the child begins to attend and by discussing their anxieties with teaching staff. Asking about the implementation of school policy with regard to teasing and bullying can help children and empower parents. Parents act as models in teaching their child how best to deal with unkind comments and intrusive staring. Working with parents directly to help them to handle difficult situations can indirectly help these children. Parents also need to know that children who are openly valued by those closest to them are also more likely to deal well with teasing.

Sometimes, brothers and sisters also become the butt of teasing particularly if they attend the same school as their sibling. Because they wish to protect the sibling and their parents from worry, they may not talk about this. In addition, siblings may be asked questions about their brother or sister, not necessarily in an unkind way but out of curiosity. This can feel just as painful to some children. They, too, can be helped by knowing how to answer these questions. They need to be included in family discussion and information about the disfigurement.

Teasing and bullying are not experienced exclusively in childhood. Increasingly, instances of bullying in the workplace are being identified. Thus, adults who acquire a visible difference in later life may experience bullying for the first time at work and may have few strategies for dealing with such problems. They may also feel that this is something they should be able to cope with themselves and be too embarrassed to discuss it. It can help to find ways of fending off the comments of others, such as joking about it, dismissing it as unimportant and/or letting others know that they have gone too far. In extreme cases, it may be necessary to complain to employers and, if the situation does not improve, to resort to the law.

Responses of teachers

'Even at that date, I was nine, I knew about "facial discrimination". I said to the teacher, "You only asked Deborah and me again because we are the two ugliest in the class"' (Kathrine, page 22).

This is a difficult area. There is research evidence that teachers may discriminate against those with a visible difference (see Section Two). Although discrimination may be expressed through blaming or the minimizing of achievements, it is also commonly expressed as overprotection and lowered expectation of the child's capabilities.

Talking with the teacher can be useful if the problem is clear-cut. However, it may be that the teacher does not recognize the problem, in which case it can be helpful for the parents to encourage the child to achieve well at school. When the child is away from school for long periods following an injury or because of hospital treatment, then extra tuition will be of benefit. This can generally be arranged in consultation with the school, who will advise on how this can be organized. If the child falls behind because of missed schooling, any problems being experienced at school can escalate.

Experience at work

Problems that can arise

Lack of confidence in taking opportunities

'... I didn't feel I could cope with such a high-profile career as this and rejected it' (Anthony, page 49).

In this situation, people with a visible difference deliberately choose a low-profile career, which makes them less noticed by others. This may be reflected in the initial choice of career, or in a reluctance to seek advancement in the chosen career. The careers service can be very useful, particularly if they offer expertise for those with special needs.

If the person has missed a lot of schooling because of hospital treatment, then his or her career path may be blighted by a lack of qualifications. The most useful intervention in this situation is direction towards appropriate training and ways of gaining further qualifications.

In addition, there may be hesitation in getting into work that requires contact with the public, or even with others in an office, a factory or in a team. Encouraging social skills and developing social coping strategies can encourage confidence to overcome this hurdle.

Lower aspirations

'I didn't encounter too much prejudice in all this, perhaps because my work was pretty low grade' (Anthony, page 50).

This cognitive and behavioural strategy minimizes the threat of prejudice by developing the belief that others will not be prejudiced if the person does not compete. It may be that the person has grown up learning to avoid competitive situations, thus reducing the fear of failure. Encouraging the person to develop his or her full potential can be helpful. This may require support in applying for jobs and promotion, further training and/or social skills work to promote effective coping in the everyday working environment.

Dating

Lack of confidence in making the initial moves

'After several weeks I want to talk to her but the difference between her beauty and my perceived ugliness and repulsiveness is too great (John, page 35).

Establishing contact can be a difficult problem for people with a visible difference, particularly for adolescents or those who may want to meet others in night-clubs and pubs. First appearances count in these settings, and the facially disfigured will be at a particular disadvantage. In addition, those people who are uncomfortable with their physical appearance are likely to be lacking in confidence and may keep to the background.

The first issue is the setting. It is likely to be easier for the person with a visible difference to make the initial move in an environment where the impact of the initial impression can be overcome. Social environments, such as youth clubs, folk clubs, sports clubs and evening classes can allow the initial contact to happen as a result of mutual activity and subsequent conversation. Getting involved in such settings may be difficult at first, but with support they can be of great value in the longer term.

It may be that lack of confidence and limited social skills are more to blame for the difficulty in forming intimate relationships than the disfigurement itself. The more the person feels generally valued and self-confident, the more likely that he or she is to feel able to form a dating relationship.

Problems in an established relationship

'... ruined intimate moments' (Jane, page 63).

Once a relationship has become established, concerns about the visible difference may cause ongoing difficulties. These problems generally relate to the person who is disfigured rather than to the partner. That person may feel ashamed of his or her appearance and may lack confidence in his or her body. Hand injuries are often associated with sexual problems, as the person may feel unable to touch or hold in an uninhibited way.

In addition, close relationships may be the forum in which unresolved grieving or anger is played out. Strong feelings of emotion can stir up old feelings of sadness that have long been buried. If the partner takes the role of a parent in the relationship, being nurturing, protective and/or critical, then the individual with the disfigurement may experience a revival of negative emotions towards that parent figure, or may become dependent and needy in response to that role.

These problems need to be understood and resolved if the relationship is to succeed. The most effective work is with the couple together. This may be appropriately carried out by an organization such as RELATE, which counsels couples who have relationship problems. The person with the visible difference may need individual work to deal with unresolved emotions. This is likely to be most successful in a psychotherapeutic setting with a therapist who is experienced in this type of approach.

Ways in which people have tried to cope

Low self-esteem leading to lack of discrimination

'In my situation, girl friends are hard to come by and it was the fear of loneliness that drove me to marry the wrong partner' (Anthony, page 50).

Sometimes, people with a visible difference have such low self-esteem that anyone who shows an interest in them becomes a likely partner. Efforts are made to cling on to that person, despite any doubts about the suitability of the match. This can lead to a succession of short-term relationships and a destructive cycle of attention and rejection. Such a pattern can be particularly problematic if it is associated with sexual promiscuity, where the individual feels that his or her only value is being sexually available.

Time spent discussing what the person wants from a relationship and discussing potential partners can encourage a belief that that person is entitled to a good relationship and has things to offer that relationship. Finding ways of overcoming the initial dating problems have already been discussed above.

Coping with treatment

Problems that can arise

Decision making about treatment

'...no-one listened to a six-year-old girl' (Kathrine, page 22).
'Plastic surgery can only go so far.... [I] do not want to take the risk of worse scars or facial paralysis' (Kathrine, pages 22–23).

The general issues relating to decision making about treatment have already been discussed in Chapter 3. Helping others to decide whether or not to have reconstructive surgery or other forms of treatment requires an understanding of the decision-making process and good communication between the clinician and those who are having treatment.

Coping with the medics and surgeons

'I remember the consultants... trailing after me in the corridors, summoning their colleagues for a look: "It's very rare that we have a case as bad as yours to treat" (Jane, page 62).

Those with a visible difference may have considerable contact with professionals. Some of the difficulties that can arise in clinics have been described in Chapter 22. This quote illustrates other types of problems the person may have to face during contact with clinicians: the unfortunate comment that is distressing and hurtful. Treating someone as a specimen whose problem is extreme can be very upsetting. The mechanism of social comparison is a useful way in which we deal with life's problems; it helps us to feel that we are not victims and that there are others who are worse off and whose problems are greater (see Moss, Chapter 18). For a person to be told that they are the worst case the professionals have seen implies victim status, and also fosters the fear that successful treatment may not be assured.

Encouraging a more positive social comparison can be useful, by identifying the positives in each case and recognizing the strengths of the individual patient. It is important for clinicians to understand the impact of their comments. Training sessions can be of great benefit, both to the quality of their clinical practice and to the patients they are treating.

Coping with the outcome of treatment

'Technically, the surgeons have done a wonderful job. I can breathe through my nostrils but I am bitterly disappointed with the aesthetic result' (John, page 33).

Treatment, particularly surgery, often carries great hopes and aspirations. The person and/or the family may anticipate that there will be great changes to appearance, and that many of the associated psychological and social problems will be resolved as a result of treatment. Sometimes there is a failure to understand the likely technical outcome of surgery. This might be because the clinician has not been clear, or perhaps because the person has only heard what he or she wants to hear. Children may expect 'magic', particularly if words such as 'this will make it better' have been used. Adults are not immune to a belief in 'magic' and their faith in the clinician may overcome a realistic appreciation of what is possible.

There are also problems associated with the process of treatment. When surgery is carried out to correct a craniofacial condition, the person may look very much worse after surgery until the swelling and bruising subside. Coping with the temporary effects of laser treatment can be difficult, for example, the reddening of the treated area and a sensitivity to make-up.

The person undergoing treatment will benefit from a clear understanding of the likely technical outcome of surgery, and also of how he or she will look during and immediately after treatment. The clinician may want to protect the patient from unnecessary worry and may appear optimistic in order to encourage the person to have the treatment. However, unrealistic expectations on the part of the patient are likely to result in distress and disappointment. Decision making needs to be in the context of knowledge of the process of treatment and the likely outcome.

The individual may benefit from support throughout this process. Coming to terms with the limitations of treatment can trigger feelings of loss and bereavement. The loss is that of the hope of great change. Effective coping with alterations in body image during and after treatment requires preparation and support throughout this process.

In conclusion

There are many diverse problems that may confront the person with a visible difference and his or her family and friends. Recognizing and understanding these problems is the first step towards developing effective ways of coping with them. Some strategies for coping have been outlined, and further detail can be found elsewhere (Bradbury, 1996). In the next chapter, case studies will be used to illustrate ways of helping in more detail.

References

Bradbury, E. T. (1996). *Counselling People with Visible Disfigurement*. Leicester: British Psychological Society.

Wheatley, C. (1993).*Puttingabravefaceonit.TheGuardian, 13November, p.17*.

Worden, J. W. (1991). *Grief Counselling and Grief Therapy*, second edition. London: Routledge.

Chapter 25

Case Studies

Nick Ambler, Eileen Bradbury and Daniela Hearst

In these three extended case studies, some of the approaches discussed above will be described in the context of an individual's story. They illustrate examples of effective care and point out where care has been ineffective or even harmful, within the context of physical treatment.

Geoff: early intervention following trauma (Nick Ambler)

When do you make a start with the psychological care of someone who has had a traumatic and disfiguring injury? Consider this:

> There has been a house fire. It began with a small explosion. No-one has been killed in the fire but Geoff, the 46-year-old owner of the house, has been seriously burned. He is rushed to the nearby general hospital where the accident and emergency consultant assesses him as burned over 32% of his body. This involves his hands and arms, face, neck and back. Within an hour, he is transferred to a specialist burns unit in another hospital. The patient is now in a critical condition.

If this man survives he will be left with extensive scars, but, at this moment, maintaining his bodily functions and preventing complications are the main priorities. In the midst of such a crisis is there really a place for thinking about his psychological care? On the face of it you might not think so. Surely any psychological issues will be swept aside by all that needs to be done for him physically?

This chapter sets out an opposing point of view. It is argued that psychological factors are involved at every stage of hospital care after a severe disfiguring injury.

A person cannot help but react to a severe or life-threatening injury. It follows that the way in which such reactions are managed will therefore have an important effect. This will influence patients' level of suffering, their behaviour, their expectations and co-operation with treatment, and also the eventual degree of recovery.

To illustrate this, we will follow Geoff's progress through hospital treatment and reflect on the psychological concerns that arise with successive stages of his care and recovery. There are two intentions behind this. The first is to try to shed some light on patients' feelings and behaviour after a serious injury. The second is to provoke some thoughts about what can be done to moderate distress and lay the foundations of a more successful long-term recovery.

Some first reactions

Geoff is now in intensive care. He has inhalation burns and it is feared that he may need to be put on a ventilator. His face and hands are extremely swollen. He is strapped to monitoring equipment and receives oxygen through a mask. He has difficulty in talking and is evidently in great pain. What he does say makes no sense and he appears to be totally confused. He is receiving morphine to relieve his pain but, before this was started, he needed to be physically restrained. Despite the morphine, there are times when he becomes frantic, especially during nursing procedures. He wrestles against the nurses and tries to get up from his bed. Sometimes he screams out: 'Get them away.'

Geoff is delirious and, but for the effects of the morphine, he would be even more agitated. However, it would be a mistake to assume that his distress is entirely due to severe pain. After surviving a delirious phase, patients sometimes describe having had a terrifying conviction of being imprisoned and then burned, knifed or tortured in some other way. Not surprisingly, this can be remembered as more frightening than the accident that caused the injuries in the first place. What then are the causes of such hallucinations?

Psychological symptoms can have a physical cause

Having inhaled poisonous fumes in the fire, it is possible that Geoff is suffering from hypoxia. This affects brain function, which in turn causes psychological disturbance. Another possibility is that the severity of his injuries has so disrupted the balance of his fluids and electrolytes as to trigger a delirious reaction. He might have suffered a metabolic encephalopathy, or perhaps he has started to develop septicaemia. Alternatively, if the dose of morphine has been reduced too rapidly, a withdrawal reaction could be the root cause of the hallucinations. Lastly, the combined physical effects of severe injury amount to a degree of shock that could also have provoked a delirious reaction.

These are the most likely explanations of this kind of psychological disturbance at this stage. There are, however, some other matters to consider.

Could a problem have existed before injury?

Serious injuries do not occur entirely randomly. There is more of a tendency for accidents to happen to people who are for some reason or another more vulnerable. Burn injuries, in particular, occur more often to the very young and the very old, or to people who are confused or unwell. For example, the effects of a condition such as epilepsy or Alzheimer's disease might have contributed to the cause of the accident. Similarly, a psychiatric illness or a drug problem may have been a factor.

Returning to our example, if it turns out that Geoff has always been a heavy drinker, then it is possible that his delirium is an effect of acute withdrawal from alcohol. Even if this was not causing hallucinations, such a dependency on alcohol and then withdrawal from this drug will almost certainly have effects on him. If the problem has not been realized, then these effects on his feelings and behaviour will appear inappropriate and a problem to manage.

Other pre-existing problems may be apparent or at least suspected. A significant number of supposed accident victims have in fact been victims of violence. Another possibility to consider is that the patient has been badly injured through a suicide attempt. The circumstances that led to this will not have been resolved and an assessment of this must therefore be brought into the plan of care. Other long-standing problems can be less clear. One example of this was a woman who became loud and aggressive, especially towards her nurses, when she needed an injection. Initially, it seemed that she had a very low tolerance of pain. Later on, however, it turned out that she had a phobia of needles. This was provoking anxiety attacks. She felt completely unable to cope with an injection and she was doing all she could to avoid it, hence the aggression.

Another important aspect of a patient's background is previous psychological stress. For example, if he or she is in the throes of a relationship break-up, a job loss, or some other personal crisis, it will not be evident from a straightforward medical history. Nevertheless, it will have a big influence on the patient's emotional state whilst in hospital.

What are the psychological reactions after trauma?

Sometimes hospital staff are surprised by how pronounced and complicated their patients' reactions can be after a serious injury. Usually a first step towards understanding such reactions is to consider what you would regard as normal in such circumstances. When a person is suddenly transported out of everyday life and confined to a hospital bed, made frail by serious injury, bombarded by severe pain, made anxious by the prospect of surgery that has an uncertain outcome, all of this having been preceded by a terrifying accident, then it is hard to imagine how this would not provoke a very distressed reaction. It also seems reasonable to assume that different people will react in different ways.

> Geoff is now out of intensive care and is in a side room in the burns unit. He still has the constant hiss of the oxygen mask at his face. He can see that his hands are in an awful mess. The nursing staff encourage him about how much better his face is looking now that the swelling has gone down but there are no mirrors for him to look and see for himself. He still suffers a lot of pain. He is still unable to move out of bed and he drifts in and out of sleep throughout the day. At times he has heavy sweats. He has periods of feeling tearful and totally depressed, sometimes for a whole day, but then the feelings lift as

mysteriously as when they descended on him. His worst moments now are when he is about to fall asleep. He has a sudden and vivid impression of the accident happening all over again. He sees his sleeves on fire and the skin peeling off his hands. All this has made Geoff worried that he may be losing his grip on reality.

Unfamiliar surroundings, constant noise, disrupted sleep, continuous pain and an inability to move around together produce sensory confusion. This would make most people at least a little disorientated and it sometimes causes hallucinations. This is sometimes called intensive care unit psychosis. This effect will have contributed to Geoff's delirium whilst he was in intensive care. At this stage, however, his delirium has resolved but he is experiencing distressing flashbacks about his accident. He may also be having anxiety attacks, which are producing the heavy sweating. For his depressed feelings to come and go as they do may seem surprising because many people would expect to feel constantly depressed in his predicament.

All of these psychological symptoms arise in such a high proportion of accident victims that they can be regarded as normal reactions. However, without advice about this, it is understandable that Geoff might be worrying about his sanity.

The way in which his mood is swinging up and down is another common reaction. It probably reflects how the full realization of what has happened is continuing gradually to unfold for him as the days pass. His feelings are still changing. In the process of this, some patients become angry. To an onlooker, this can seem completely out of place, especially if the anger is directed at a close relative or at nurses. In contrast, some patients can seem unaware of the seriousness of their injuries, behaving cheerfully and joking as if to say, 'I have pulled through and I will be fit again in a few days' time'. Others become anxious and needy, making constant demands of their nurses in a way that seems immature and unreasonable.

These differing reactions are what some would call psychological defences; they are varying but characteristic ways of behaving after a personal crisis. There is no way of predicting exactly how any single person is going to react but in most cases the reaction is one that evolves rather than remains static. Sometimes a patient's reaction after trauma will seem odd or even alarming. Even so, it is rarely the case that a psychological reaction cannot, at least, be safely contained.

What can be done to help?

It has been put to me more than once that of course patients get distressed, understandably so, but there really is not much one can do to help. Could Geoff's care have been improved so far and if so, how?

Several things might have given him more of a sense of composure and control during his ordeal. In the first few days after the accident, some frequent prompts about where he was, the time of day, and what was happening would all have helped to give him some sense of *orientation*. Even though he might still have been only fleetingly alert, such simple prompting would have helped to calm him between the terrifying hallucinations.

Later on there was room for improvement in the level of *explanation* provided. Had time been set aside to talk to him about psychological reactions to trauma, then some of the symptoms would have seemed more normal to him and he would not have worried about his sanity.

Geoff's pattern of *sleep* was chaotic. As his recovery progressed, he could have been encouraged to avoid daytime dozing in order to get better sleep at night. Establishing a regular cycle improves the quality of sleep and helps with orientation.

The problem of *flashbacks* and *nightmares* can be so vivid and frightening that a person will do anything to stay awake. If someone is drinking numerous cups of strong coffee or is pacing the hospital corridors at night it could simply be an attempt to avoid another nightmare. Sometimes, during a distressed phase, some patients repeatedly go missing from the hospital ward because of fear about how flashbacks or other reactions have appeared to take them over. Sedating medication can help to overcome this, but it is not an entirely reliable method. It is helpful to tackle the fear of flashbacks and nightmares through, for example, guidance about how best to calm down after one has occurred. This restores a sense of control. It helps the person to confront the problem rather than becoming caught up in the exhausting process of trying to avoid frightening reminders of the accident.

When is the trauma finished?

It may be a mistake to regard the accident as the only trauma endured by a patient. So far in our example, Geoff's hallucinations and flashbacks have also been a terrifying experience and there is more to come.

Geoff has full thickness burns on his hands and on some parts of his face. He has already undergone skin grafting, taking donor skin from the tops of his thighs, but there will be more operations. He openly says how frightened he feels about further surgery. However, the next distressing event occurs during bathing. It is now that he catches first sight of himself in a mirror. He cries uncontrollably for an hour afterwards. He then withdraws into himself and refuses to see anyone. At night, he spends two hours in tearful conversation with one of the night nurses. The next day he asks to talk to someone about his feelings. The registrar in plastic surgery comes to see him and offers him medication to lift his mood and help him to sleep.

There is an issue here about the *management of pain*. So far, medication has been the only form of help provided. At this stage, he is probably getting two levels of pain relief. The first will be a regular dose to help him to cope with the constant pain from his wounds. The second level is a top-up before any kind of procedure, such as a change of dressings.

There are two complications about pain relief that can easily be overlooked. First, people vary in how they respond to their medication. The only way properly to take account of this is to monitor the level of pain using a standardized patient self-rating measure. Most hospitals have a pain management service or a pain clinic that can advise about this. Other methods of assessing pain are notoriously unreliable, especially those that rely entirely on the judgements made by care staff.

The second complication is that people also vary in their capacity to cope with different levels of pain. Consider, for example, how composed some patients are about painful procedures compared with those who become very agitated even before the procedure begins. The ability to cope with pain will be strongly influenced by the beliefs a person has about it. For example, someone who understands the procedure as being helpful and who is relaxed beforehand is better able to tolerate pain than someone who regards the procedure as frightening and unnecessary.

In Geoff's case, he could be helped with better preparation. As he begins a regimen of hand exercises to prevent contractures, it will help him if he understands what contractures are, why they occur, and how the exercises work. He needs to be asked both how *able* he feels to cope with the pain and *how* he tries to cope with it. Many people use distraction, diverting attention in some other direction as best they can. Sometimes, albeit less often, a patient needs to have some sense of control, say through taking a lead with a procedure, calling for breaks in it, perhaps even rating his or her own performance at the end. Some professional helpers find this difficult to accept, perhaps reflecting a similar need in themselves to be in control.

Another concern of some professionals is the possibility of inducing a long-term addiction to medication. In fact, this rarely arises, yet such a concern could mean a patient receives insufficient pain relief.

If problems in relation to pain cannot be resolved by medication and advice about coping methods, then this is the point at which referral to a pain specialist should be considered. To overlook such an important issue could prolong an unnecessary degree of suffering.

There is another important issue regarding the *management of emotional distress*. Geoff has been offered medication to control his distress. This can also be a contentious issue amongst hospital staff. On one side there is an argument that, if a person is still overcoming a state of shock, progressively coming to terms with the effects of injury, then the process should not be stifled by antidepressants or tranquillizers. This would arguably impair the process of adjustment. Brief counselling as an alternative could help to move the process forward and hence be a much more useful way of resolving such distress.

There are, however, some quite different circumstances in which such a position is too rigid. For example, where a patient is strongly requesting medication as a kind of prop, this can help them to cope with a situation that they are otherwise finding intolerable. Alternatively, again in relation to pain, when a procedure is provoking extreme tension, then medication can help to reduce the anxiety.

Between these separate positions there is debate and a judgement to be made about whether or not medication is an appropriate and helpful method of managing psychological distress at the time of acute injury. In other circumstances, when a patient appears to be psychiatrically disturbed or in the throes of a prolonged withdrawal reaction, then referral to a specialist is necessary.

Confronting the appearance of injuries

In Geoff's case, there has been quite a wait before he eventually sees his facial injuries. There does seem to be a consensus that after facial burns it is better to wait several days at least before the first encounter with a mirror. During this time, there is usually a substantial improvement as swelling recedes and it is thought that an earlier look in the mirror is unnecessarily distressing. There also seems to be a consensus that the 'first look' in a mirror should be sensitively managed, allowing time, privacy and moral support with the company of one of the nursing team. Taking the trouble to do this allows a proper exploration of injuries rather than a fleeting look.

This is perhaps the most carefully thought through stage in the psychological management of disfiguring injuries. Nevertheless, there are some aspects that are not always considered. First, the absence of mirrors in a room does not necessarily prevent some people from catching sight of themselves in other ways. A window gives a fairly good reflection with darkness outside and there are other reflective surfaces that come into sight. It is possible to borrow a make-up mirror from a relative. Unprepared and unsupported, the shock of a first look in this way leads some to avoid or deny their injuries thereafter.

The same problem arises for others who, without ever having caught sight of their injuries, go to great lengths to avoid ever seeing them. This does not just apply to facial wounds but can be for any part of the body. It is not too difficult to avoid looking at any injury if it is usually dressed with bandages or covered in some other way.

How might this best be handled?

My own view is that this situation is less likely to arise if the process of psychological care for disfiguring injuries begins at an earlier stage. After all, even without the use of the mirror, a patient will from the start be building up a picture of what the injuries might look like, probably with associated fears and expectations. This is influenced by the remarks made to them by their doctors and nurses and by the first reactions of their visitors.

A more thorough approach would be to provide information about facial or other injuries from the outset. This includes how their appearance is likely to change over the coming days and, if there are no mirrors around, the reasons for this. Agreeing on a time to be set aside for looking over facial or other injuries after these have started to settle should give some reassurance. It emphasizes that it is regarded as an important stage and that there will be plenty of opportunity to ask questions and clarify things. It helps to side-step the possibility that the patient will go on avoiding the 'first look' or stumble on it without support or preparation. In Geoff's case, this did not happen and he was left guessing, probably matching the damage he could see on his hands to the likely appearance of his face. When he eventually saw himself in a mirror, there was nothing to soften the blow, or to help him pick himself up until some time later.

Are there any other sources of psychological stress?

- When Geoff's sister heard of the accident she came straight over to be with him. She spends the day-time at his bedside, then rushes home to sort out her children, and then back to the hospital again for the evening.
- The police suspect that an intruder deliberately started the fire in Geoff's house and they want him to make a statement.
- This was the second fire on Geoff's estate in recent weeks and several national newspapers have asked for an interview.
- Geoff's insurers want to send someone to interview him about the accident.
- A group of friends from work are planning to come up and see him and surprise him with cards and presents.
- Geoff's personnel manager has been in touch to arrange a visit to talk over his plans to return to work.
- On one occasion, both his mother and his ex-wife arrived at the same time for a visit. They ended up having a row with each other at his bedside.

There is an accumulation of stresses here. The most obvious is that over-whelming numbers of visitors are tiring. Also, a relative who carries out a bedside vigil can cause them both to become exhausted.

A situation such as this really needs someone to take a lead in containing all these pressures. This means working out with the patient about how much company feels right, organizing visitors and holding back other unwanted outside pressures. It may only require a hint or a simple observation to prompt a close relative to take up this role.

It is inevitable that Geoff will have to explain his accident to friends and family, helpers and others. The process of recounting an accident is often tiring and upsetting. Having to tell the whole story repeatedly to different people is even more exhausting and it would help Geoff if he were able to work out a short version of what happened. It would also help for him to know how to change the subject tactfully as a way of avoiding having to go over the story time and again.

A widely publicized story on television and in the newspapers is not necessarily a bad thing for an accident victim. Certainly, all the attention can be a huge distraction, which will affect the otherwise unfolding process of adjustment to the injury. Being pursued by reporters is stressful, then finding basic mistakes in the way an accident is publicly reported can be upsetting.

On the other hand, accident victims are often portrayed in heroic terms by the media and this can give quite a boost. Later on, being easily recognized and having the story of the accident widely known can be quite an advantage for someone with disfiguring injuries. It reduces the sometimes rude and intrusive questioning from other people, even from complete strangers. Rather than walk up and demand to know what happened, they may have something different and more encouraging to say if they already know the story from a newspaper.

Another reflection on Geoff's situation concerns the cause of his accident. Having been the likely victim of an arson attack, and with the perpetrator still at large, his hospital bed will seem like an exposed and vulnerable place to be. Geoff might be understandably afraid of receiving an especially unwanted visitor.

The row that took place at Geoff's bedside is by no means an unusual event. It may seem astonishing that tensions within families can spill out in this way at the very time when an injured person most needs stability and support. It happens nevertheless. Perhaps it is easier to understand why this arises if some of the following also apply. First, the shock of the near-death of a loved one inevitably has an effect on close relatives as well as on the patient. Although many relatives seem composed and clear-thinking, it is understandable that some are emotional and seemingly irrational at this time. They now face worries about the future. There may be recriminations about the way the accident occurred. There is probably stress at home because of all that needs to be sorted out. Close relationships might already have been strained. An accident is an important family event and will often bring warring factions together in the same room. These different ingredients can form a volatile mixture, affecting the patient and also professional helpers. Added to this is the fact that another frequent psychological effect of trauma on a patient is anger or quick temper. This only magnifies tensions that may have existed between the patient and a spouse or others in the family.

How can this be managed?

As a rule, this is not a time to try to resolve marital conflicts, or to embark on any kind of family therapy. This applies at least until the acute phase of injury has passed by. Such conflicts need to be contained or set aside. If some kind of help is required to sort out family problems then this could be arranged, but it should begin at a later stage. If a particular relative needs help, this might also be set up now, but carried out away from the hospital ward. Geoff does not need extra stress from his relatives. He should not have to keep the peace between them. He needs to be able to concentrate his energies on his recovery.

Approaching discharge

Geoff has been told he can go home in three days' time. He has already had two successful weekends at his sister's home. He is really cheerful and looking forward to seeing his newly repaired house again. He realizes that he will be coming back to hospital for further operations later on but this is far from his mind now. Basically, he cannot wait to get back and resume a normal everyday life.

In a specialist unit, everyone seems accustomed to disfigurement. There is little natural preparation for the reactions of strangers in the outside world. This protective effect has been described as a 'cocoon' experience. After returning home, to suddenly be confronted with the unpleasantness of other people's reactions to disfiguring injuries can turn a confident person into a virtual recluse. If there are going to be problems with other people's reactions then it would be advisable to moderate the impact by confronting these gradually before discharge home. A programme of accompanied trips, first, around the hospital and then elsewhere, will gradually dismantle any 'cocoon' effect. It helps to prevent a situation where someone is discharged from hospital not realizing what effect their altered appearance will have in everyday life and, when they do, finding that there is no-one around to help them to come to terms with this.

Another problem that may be awaiting Geoff relates to his long-term expectations. In the early stages of recovery, appearance improves quickly. Successful surgery will have boosted his confidence with a leap forward after each operation. With things changing so quickly and possibly a misunderstanding about what can ultimately be achieved with plastic surgery, people in Geoff's situation can easily build up completely unrealistic hopes about how much they will regain of their previous appearance. Geoff may well be thinking to himself: 'Alright, I don't look so good at the moment but I will look much better later after more surgery.' If so, he may feel he has no need to worry about making any adjustments. He might well decide simply to avoid people for the time being and to wait until he regains an appearance similar to the way he looked before the accident.

If not checked, these false hopes can continue after discharge home. It may be, however, that no-one will want to confront this with him. It is uncomfortable breaking bad news to someone by dashing their hopes about the future. This might seem unnecessary, especially in view of the fact that it is not possible to know, at a relatively early stage in recovery, what the long-term appearance of scars is likely to be. Nevertheless, it is possible to check that a person's expectations are realistic rather than to allow false hopes to build up and then suddenly be dashed later. The real pay-off from this will come at some point in the future. The eventual outcome of Geoff's surgery will be measured, in his eyes at least, by the extent to which he feels able to regain his self-confidence and resume his everyday life despite his changed appearance.

Conclusions and future directions

During the course of his hospital care, Geoff has made a good recovery from life-threatening injuries. This traumatic experience brought out different phases of psychological distress in him. This description covered only the most visible and obvious aspects of his distress. Had Geoff been severely injured in some way other than by burns, the account of his reactions might well have followed the same pattern.

There is a contrast between the way Geoff's psychological distress was managed and the possible alternatives. What he received was a *passive* regimen of psychological care. That is to say that his psychological reactions were observed but the only stages at which help was offered were those when his distress or behaviour became extreme.

The alternatives are not complicated. They involve: information and explanation; prompting to improve his orientation and sleep; some containment of outside pressures; advanced preparation for the stressful stages, including operations and confronting disfigurement; individually tailored pain management; and preparation for the problems that may arise after discharge. It is also necessary to be clear when other specialists should be consulted regarding pain and psychological reactions. This is a *proactive* regimen of psychological care.

To set up a proactive regimen takes several steps. It requires building up a knowledge base amongst staff about the causes of psychological symptoms, covering physiological, psychological and pre-existing factors. The next steps are to work out when and how to intervene, and then to decide who will be responsible for this. Another step is to arrange an effective liaison with the psychological and pain specialists who are sometimes needed; without preparation, it is difficult to know how to get the best out of their consultations.

All of this takes time and organization, but the pay-offs should be considerable: it will reduce the suffering of patients, it should empower nursing staff in the psychological aspects of their work, it builds greater trust with and co-operation by patients, and it paves the way for a better long-term adjustment to disfiguring injuries.

This account has covered the basic and straightforward aspects of psychological care with severe injury. There is presently considerable research interest in stress reactions after trauma, which addresses the reasons why it is that some people cope well while others get into difficulties. This research promises a great deal for guiding in more detail the early management of people in a similar predicament to Geoff.

Finally, what happens next for Geoff? It is unlikely that he will have any complaints about his hospital care; it saved his life. Nevertheless, it could have been better. As he leaves hospital, his future prospects are uncertain. There is a good chance that he will adapt well, overcoming his traumatic experience and restoring his everyday life, but there is also a significant risk that it will not go so well for him. If so, he may look back and wonder why things could not have been managed a little better whilst he was still in hospital.

Mary: facial cancer, disease and disfigurement (Eileen Bradbury)

Sometimes, the work in this field presents with several problems at once. For those with head and neck cancer, the issues relate both to the cancer and to the disfigurement that follows treatment.

Mary is a 54-year-old lady who has worked for many years as a nursing auxiliary in a psychiatric hospital. She has a son aged 30 and a daughter aged 24. Her relationship with her husband, a businessman, has been quite unhappy for the last few years as she feels they have been growing apart. Mary and her husband, Andy, have always drunk alcohol regularly, but Mary had started to drink more heavily, using alcohol to numb the pain of her increasing unhappiness with her marriage. She smokes 20 cigarettes a day.

She is close to her daughter who lives down the road. Her mother is still alive, but growing increasingly forgetful; Mary calls in most days to check that she is coping. Mary and her husband have a small circle of mutual friends. Her main confidante is a particular friend whom she has known since childhood. She has no sisters or brothers and little social contact with colleagues at work.

In October, Mary went on a routine visit to the dentist for a check-up. For some time she had been troubled by a persistent ulcer on one side of her jaw. The dentist suggested that she should see her family doctor. She felt that the problem was too trivial for this and continued for some time with pastilles from the chemist. When she visited her doctor for another problem some months later, she mentioned the ulcer to him. He told her that it was probably nothing to worry about, but it might be worth having it checked by a specialist at the hospital. He referred her to a consultant at the cancer hospital. For the first time, Mary began to worry. Until then, cancer had not crossed her mind. However, she was reassured by the doctor's unconcerned manner, and she had always been good at ignoring difficulties in the hope that they would go away. She cancelled her first appointment because of a social event at work. It was February of the year following the visit to the dentist when she finally attended the outpatient clinic.

Mary's response to early suspicions was typical of her; she coped by denying the problem and used the reactions of the medical professionals to reinforce that denial. This caused her to delay her treatment. It would have been appropriate for both the dentist and the doctor to be more specific and to make clear their concerns, but many professionals are reluctant to frighten their patients. These two did not frighten Mary, and they failed to pass on information in a clear way that would have confronted her denying response and ensured that she sought early help.

She sat in the clinic waiting-room with her husband. He had offered to come with her, although she would have preferred her daughter to come. She looked around her and saw people with faces disfigured by swelling and surgery, some had missing eyes, others had tracheostomy holes in their necks. The atmosphere was muted and rather fearful. She felt a fraud, coming with such a trivial complaint. She wanted to get the consultation over with as quickly as possible. When her turn came, she went into a consulting room full of people in white coats. She sat opposite the surgeon, who took a brief history and then examined her mouth and felt her neck. He told her that the ulcer was suspicious, and she would need to come into hospital so that they could take a sample for analysis. The surgeon made it clear that there was urgency and that she should be admitted next week. Although Mary missed much of the detail because she was preoccupied with the uncomfortable feeling of being watched and was feeling very anxious, Andy understood much of what the surgeon said. When they went home, she did not want to talk about it. Against the advice of the surgeon, she continued to smoke and drink.

Mary was admitted the following week and, under a light general anaesthetic, a biopsy was taken from her mouth. She returned to the clinic to see the surgeon a fortnight later. The news was bad; the 'ulcer' had been diagnosed as a malignant tumour and needed to be removed as a matter of urgency. The surgeon said she should come into hospital in the next week and he would remove the tumour together with the surrounding tissue and bone. He would have to replace the bone from her jaw with bone from her rib. He emphasized once more that she must stop smoking and drinking, and told her that, if she continued to smoke, the flap might fail. When her husband asked what had caused the tumour, the surgeon said he could not be sure, but that smoking and drinking were risk factors. After the consultation, she and her husband were invited to spend a short time in a quiet side room with the psychologist who attended the clinic. They were encouraged to ask questions and to clarify anything they wanted to know. The psychologist asked them about family and friends and suggested that other people liked to help at times like this. Practicalities such as the care of Mary's mother were also discussed. Andy became tearful but Mary felt numb; it had not sunk in. The word 'malignant' kept going round in her head and she heard little else. However, she was moved by Andy's reaction. He comforted and supported her and took it upon himself to tell their children and her close friend, who all gave her support over the days before the operation. She was very worried about her mother, and Andy arranged for their daughter to take over that contact for the time being.

The telling of bad news is very difficult for the professional, but the way in which it is done is of profound importance. There are certain guidelines that are helpful:

• Sit down and talk to the person face to face (not standing looking down at an examination couch).
• Try to ensure that a close relative or friend is there to support the patient and to hear what is being said; the anxious patient finds it hard to take in all the information.
• Give the information in a clear way using nontechnical language.
• Make sure that it has been understood by checking with the patient or relative.
• It can be helpful to give written information. Some clinicians tape the consultation and give the patient a copy of the tape; this has been found to increase the amount of information remembered and to reduce anxiety.

Hearing bad news is very difficult for the patient. It takes time to absorb the information. Early responses commonly include feelings of numbness, unreality and denial, which are all manifestations of shock. For people like Mary, who commonly cope by denial and avoidance, these responses become magnified. Of crucial importance is having someone close to support her, to attend appointments with her, and to help her to come to terms with the information. We all need to cling to hope; selective listening can help that feeling of optimism. However, it is helpful to give the patient and the supporter a quiet period of time after the diagnosis to work through early fears and to clarify information.

Mary's husband has played a very important role. He listened to the information, asked questions to ensure that he understood, supported Mary, and mobilized her family and other forms of social support. However, like Mary, he is likely to be under great strain at this time, and it may be that it is he, more than Mary, who needs professional help in order to help his wife. Although they have had marital difficulties, this situation has drawn them together.

In terms of Mary's responses, this is not the time to confront her denial. This could be very threatening to her and make it harder for her to cope. However, any questions should be answered honestly. If she did not want to know the answer, she would not ask the question.

Mary went into hospital for the operation. She was in the operating theatre for most of the day. When she came back to the ward, Andy was shocked by her appearance, as her face was swollen and distorted following radical surgery. She spent a few days in a specialized high dependency unit connected to drips and monitors. This gave Andy time to look at her and get used to her appearance. He realized the extent of the problem for the first time, and found himself becoming angry with the staff if he felt they were not caring for her every need. He felt guilty about his behaviour towards her in the past and this turned to anger. He was also angry that she had cancer. The staff found him rather difficult and tended to avoid him.

Andy's responses at this time were a reflection of past history, his own feelings of guilt and the grieving reaction to the cancer. It would have been helpful if a member of staff had spent time with him to try to understand his feelings. This would have made it easier to offer him the support he needed. His daughter was busy with her grandmother and he was in particular need of psychological support. Offering help at this time, whilst Mary was unable to talk, would help to prepare him for the times ahead when she will need his support.

Mary gradually came round and was moved to the general ward. She was relieved that the operation was over. She tried not to look at her face in a mirror and believed that her appearance would soon improve. The biggest problem in the early days was to do with swallowing; she found it very difficult to swallow anything. She did not like hospital food, so Andy brought her food in from home. Although it was light and very liquid, she had enormous difficulty in eating it. The surgeon and the speech and language therapist could find no reason for this. Andy was getting increasingly frustrated with her and old tensions began to surface. Mary became tearful and showed signs of depression. She became withdrawn, often flat in her mood and lethargic, and had difficulty with sleeping. The psychologist then spent time with her. Mary felt that Andy was trying to control her and she felt resistant to this. She described feelings of anger towards Andy, but did not want to think about her situation in more general terms. The psychologist encouraged her to explore her feelings, and Mary talked for the first time about her fears of cancer, and particularly of being disfigured. She became very emotional and the psychologist listened and encouraged her to talk. She helped Mary to understand her responses to Andy and helped her to reframe the problem, shifting it from a battle over feeding to a need to regain some feelings of control. They agreed ways in which she could control her own eating by strategies such as privacy and plenty of time. The psychologist then talked with both Andy and Mary, and helped to draw some of the heat from the situation. She also agreed to spend more time with Mary talking through the fears she had raised about her illness and also her fears about disfigurement.

It is vital to understand the factors that are affecting behaviour. Old patterns of interaction and styles of coping influence responses to new threats and stressful situations. It is of particular importance to facilitate communication between the patient and those who will be responsible for care. The intervention should be based on individual need and be offered to whichever party needs it at any given time.

Depression following major surgery for head and neck cancer is common. It may be a short-term reaction to the difficulties of the situation. For some, it becomes a more prolonged and disabling condition. Referral to a psychiatrist for assessment and antidepressant medication can be useful when the client shows signs of severe depression. As alcohol and cigarettes are high-risk factors in this group, withdrawal symptoms can compound the problems.

Mary was eventually discharged home. Andy had to be at work during the day and arranged for her to be visited by friends. Their daughter also called regularly. Mary was aware that friends were shocked by her appearance when they first saw her, but they reassured her that it would improve and that surgeons 'can work miracles'. Her psychological care was taken over by a counsellor from her local general practice, who had discussed the situation with the psychologist from the hospital. The counsellor encouraged Mary to continue to talk openly about her feelings. She felt reasonably happy at this time, but continued to postpone going out, always finding an excuse. She had been asked to go to a social event at work but did not go, leaving home only for hospital appointments. She applied for early retirement.

The counsellor discussed with Mary her fears of going out. Mary felt that she did not want to be seen by people who had known her before, as they would be shocked and would feel sorry for her. She felt that strangers would know that she had had cancer and she found this idea disturbing. She felt that she had lost her privacy and that everyone had access to her worst fears. For a long time, hopes of some miraculous improvement in her appearance had allowed her to postpone going out, but, as time went by, she came to realize that there were no miracles and that she would remain disfigured. This realization became final at the last visit to the surgeon, who told her that there was little more that could be done surgically. The surgeon clearly felt that he had achieved a good result. Mary's family and friends told her that she was lucky that she had not died and that her face was not too bad. Mary did not feel lucky and became confused about her responses. She felt that she was not entitled to make a fuss. She had seen people much worse than herself in the clinic and had known that others had not survived. She agreed that her disfigurement was not now particularly great, but her face was altered and she still found it hard to recognize herself in the mirror. She studied her face for long periods, searching for her old self. All this triggered a grieving response as she mourned the loss of her old appearance. She became angry and also very tearful, but only expressed her feelings with the counsellor as she did not want to upset her family who were so pleased with her progress. She felt that it was not fair, but also felt a sense of personal responsibility because of her drinking and smoking, and because she had postponed her visit to the doctor. This caused her to turn her anger in on herself, putting her at risk for a further bout of depression.

The counsellor helped her to talk through these issues and recognize that she had been responding to the situation in which she found herself, rather than taking deliberate action to increase the risk. Mary also knew that she would avoid excessive alcohol and smoking in the future and would take more care of her general health. She was able to 'forgive' herself. She also came to realize that it was easier in the end to feel that there was a cause, because this allowed her to have a sense of control over future events. Many people develop a generalized anxiety and become hypervigilant to any symptoms when they do not know the cause of the cancer.

There are important issues to consider here. Mary's acceptance of her altered appearance was postponed by the clinic visits and the hopes for further surgery. Her grieving could only begin when she let go of those hopes. However, this grieving was complicated by the opinion expressed by others that she was lucky to be alive and lucky not to have a major disfigurement. She did not feel lucky, and, whilst this approach may have helped her family and friends to cope, it did not help her and made her angry. She felt she was not entitled to her emotions and thus felt isolated and unsupported. It would have been useful for the counsellor to have talked with Mary, her husband and her daughter, to allow these feelings to be communicated. This would have helped to empower the family to support each other, thus shifting their reliance on support away from the counsellor.

Mary was then able to work with the counsellor on coping strategies for going out and meeting people. She was asked to grade the difficulty of specific situations. For example, Mary felt that the easiest would be going to the local shop where they did not know her well, whereas the hardest would be to go to a social event relating to her husband's work. She also felt that it would be difficult to walk down a busy shopping street, but felt she could go out in a group with friends who had already seen her face. Having arranged for her to go to the shop with her daughter, Mary was worried about what to say if anyone asked her what had happened. She discussed with the counsellor what she would like to say, and rehearsed the explanation that she had had an operation but she was now better. She knew she did not want to talk about the cancer, and so decided she would add: 'I don't want to talk about it'. Mary found that no-one at the shop asked anything, but she was conscious of stares. She discussed later how anxious this made her feel: beating heart, sweatiness and feelings of panic. She almost wished they had asked, so that she could give her responses. The counsellor felt it would be useful for her to deal with her physical feelings of anxiety and taught her breathing control: steady breathing, concentrating on breathing out and letting go with every exhalation. She also explained how to control muscular tension by sitting and standing in a more relaxed way. Her daughter sat in on this discussion so that she could help her mother subsequently.

The counsellor also explained that people might stare because they could not at first work out what was wrong with Mary's face and that they were curious, but also rather embarrassed. She suggested that Mary had three main choices: to ignore the staring, to divert her attention, or to confront people. Mary did not want to do the last of these as she felt too vulnerable. They discussed how she could ignore the reactions by unfocusing her eyes so that she did not see people looking, and how she could distract herself with other activities or thoughts. Mary needed to practise the breathing and relaxation techniques to help her to do this. Another visit to the shop was planned and this time Mary felt it went much better. She was able to control her panic, to busy herself and to talk about other things. She felt more in control of the situation, which gave her confidence to continue this work.

In the meantime, Mary's personal life had not stood still. She had been to see her mother and found that she coped well with the change to her face. Mary was then able to resume the role of helping her mother, although she accepted Andy's suggestion of having a Home Help as well. She and Andy found that the situation had drawn them closer together. The fear of death had made him realize how much he loved her, and his support made her feel loved and made him feel needed. Friends were also supportive and she drew closer to them. Thus, the family and social network helped her to cope.

In this context of optimism and support, Mary made good progress in becoming used to dealing with exposure to social situations. She gained in confidence, and learned to recognize and understand the responses of others. However, she still found it hard to go out on her own, preferring to have someone with her. She also avoided formal occasions when everyone was dressed up; she felt she could not look attractive and this made her feel uncomfortable. She still felt sad when she saw herself in the mirror.

The counsellor worked with her on her feelings of unattractiveness and 'difference'. In talking these issues through, Mary realized that she continued to feel pitied because of the cancer. She was encouraged to see herself as a survivor, not a victim, but as someone who had been brave and had come through. This allowed her to accept what her friends and family had been saying all along. She found she could hold her head up and feel proud of herself, that her scars were a mark of courage and survival, not of disease and death. As she learned to attribute a different meaning to her scars, she was able to recover emotionally and to live her life in a more fulfilling way. She was retired early on the grounds of ill health and enjoyed her retirement. The counsellor and all other professionals withdrew.

An important aim of psychological help is to encourage a return to normality. By involving the family in the work and by empowering Mary to cope, the counsellor facilitated the transition from Mary's status as patient to that of a normal member of the community. After all she had been through, Mary was now stronger emotionally than she had been before, and had learned that she could cope and that she was loved.

Mary was fortunate in that she received specialist psychological help both in hospital and following discharge. This type of help is not widely available and too often people such as Mary and her family are left to cope by themselves.

Tamsin: the baby born with a congenital craniofacial condition: parental adjustment to the birth (Daniela Hearst)

Tamsin, aged 4 years, the second child of professional parents, Ann and Michael, has Crouzon's syndrome. She was born with premature fusion of the small joints between the various skull and facial bones, giving her a spherical appearance. She had shallow, underdeveloped orbits, so her eyes were extremely prominent and bulging. Her mid-face was recessed, making her nose look beaky. As a result of her abnormal facial anatomy, her upper airway was narrow, causing breathing and associated feeding difficulties. When introduced to her new sister, the older child remarked, 'Mummy, she looks just like ET'.

Tamsin was two weeks old when she and her parents made the three-and-a-half-hour journey to the craniofacial unit of a specialist children's hospital. The older sister remained with relatives. A series of investigations and consultations followed. Ann and Michael attended the consultations. The psychologist introduced herself and was told in no uncertain terms that everything was fine and her visits were not required or welcome.

Tamsin was a fretful, irritable baby who struggled to suck. Breast feeding had been abandoned and even the bottle had to be replaced with a nasogastric tube. Ann and Michael appeared shell-shocked; they asked questions but appeared not to hear the replies. They sat for long hours looking at Tamsin but rarely held her or talked to her.

In the following days, Ann became increasingly angry, complaining bitterly about the inefficiency and discomfort of hospital life. She was sick of the endless waiting, the lack of information given and the quality of help offered. She felt she was in a goldfish bowl, under permanent scrutiny, with staff coming in and out unasked, disturbing Tamsin while not offering the practical help Ann required. Michael seemed shrouded in a veil of misery and rarely spoke. The nurses noticed their own reluctance to enter the cubicle other than when absolutely necessary. They felt deskilled and talked of Ann and Michael as 'difficult parents'.

After a particularly trying morning spent waiting for eye and ear tests that gave inconclusive results, Ann told the ward staff nurse that as nothing was being done for Tamsin, they might as well take her home. She declared her extreme dissatisfaction with the hospital and threatened to make a formal complaint. The psychologist, who was witness to this, commiserated with her anger and how out of control everything might feel. Ann burst into tears, pouring out her despair and frustration, while Michael sat beside her, struggling with his tears.

It was all such a shock, Ann said. Everything had gone so devastatingly wrong. The birth had been long and complicated, the baby was whisked off and Ann thought she had died. She heard someone say 'syndrome' and immediately thought her child had Down's syndrome. Her first sight of Tamsin shocked her terribly and for two days she could hardly bring herself to look at or touch the child. She said she felt numb with horror and found herself thinking: 'I wish I had a real baby'. Now, at a second hospital, far from home and her other child, she felt out of her depth. Would Tamsin end up as a cabbage? Who would ever want to play with her? What could surgery do for her? Michael said he knew it was no-one's fault, but he could not stop blaming himself somehow. They had never heard of Crouzon's syndrome and were desperate for information, but complained that the doctors seemed hesitant to say anything. 'It's as if they feel we won't be able to handle it. Why don't they realize it's the *not* knowing that's the worst of all.'

Here, it seemed, the thoughts and feelings of the past and the present were being expressed. Ann and Michael's expectations had been confounded; they had suffered loss of the 'normal' baby they had anticipated and needed to grieve. Yet, how could they do this, while dealing with the current anxieties and uncertainties surrounding Tamsin and the implications for the future? Far from home, in yet another hospital, and cut off from family and community, where was the 'space' for them to express the anger, shame and disappointment at not producing a perfect baby? It was not surprising that some of that anger should be displaced on to the hospital. It was important for Ann and Michael to be able to talk over the events and feelings of the birth, and, in particular, to be allowed to be angry and attribute blame, however unfounded. They were still in a state of shock and disbelief – a barrier to absorbing new information about Tamsin – while terrified about what her future would hold.

Hospital 'expertise' can also be experienced as others knowing better about your child; Ann and Michael badly needed to feel back in control and regain their feelings of competence as parents. As well as being listened to *and heard*, they required the provision of written source information about Crouzon's syndrome. Once provided, the literature could be read, discussed and absorbed by the parents at their own pace. As their knowledge grew, so did their optimism and their ability to absorb the answers to their questions. The term 'syndrome' lost some of its frightening connotations.

Life on the ward improved for all when a better balance between the need for privacy and care giving was negotiated between the parents and the nurses. Here again was the issue of parental control – much at risk when the hospital system dictated the boundaries (the threatened formal complaint was never made).

As Ann talked about the birth, she began to share her reactions to Tamsin's appearance, in particular, her dread that she would never feel as close to this baby as she did to her first child. Outright neglect and rejection is rare, but mother–baby interaction (including face to face contact, verbal communication and smiling) is often reduced when the baby is disfigured. Slowly, as Ann gained confidence in looking after Tamsin, which included learning how to feed her by nasogastric tube, she began to notice the things Tamsin was beginning to do and thus began to experience her as a recognizable person, not just a bundle of facial abnormalities. Michael became expert at the practical issues surrounding Tamsin's care. He preferred not to share his thoughts and feelings with professional staff, a decision that was important to respect, while ensuring that the opportunity for discussion was always available.

The investigations on Tamsin were now complete. Immediate surgery was proposed to alleviate the pressure inside her skull. It was also confirmed that she had a narrowing of the upper airway, which was causing breathing problems. Ann and Michael were desperate to return home to 'touch base', and see their other daughter. An operation was booked for a week hence.

Tamsin was eight weeks old when she underwent her first major surgery. It was a success, but many physical difficulties remained. Three weeks later, she required the insertion of a nasal prong to aid her breathing, followed by an examination of her ears under anaesthetic. Her eyes were so protruding, they tended to pop out when she became distressed or angry; Ann and Michael became adept at putting them back in each time. All in all, in her first two years, Tamsin had eight hospital admissions, including two major operations to remodel her skull, to protect her eyes and to save her vision. At the age of two years, Tamsin was of fragile physique but with a forceful personality. Despite moderate deafness in both ears, she reached out to the world about her, was eager to explore, play and show and receive affection. Ann and Michael appeared delighted with and by her. Despite the nasal prong, she still had impaired breathing, particularly at night, which resulted in repeated chest infections. Of particular concern was the potential effect of chronically lowered oxygen saturation on her general health and mental development.

There were difficult decisions to be made. Tamsin could be offered surgery to advance her mid-face and thereby increase the size of her air passages. This would involve a very major and complex procedure with all the attendant risks. Tamsin was still very young, not physically strong, and had already had two lengthy operations. There was a real threat to her survival and no guarantee that the breathing problems would be solved. To delay surgery, however, could seriously affect her physical and intellectual development.

Ann and Michael had several long meetings with the doctors, ending in angry frustration on both sides. The parents wanted to know every step and technical detail of the planned procedure and complained that information was being withheld. The surgeons felt that they could not be any more explicit without requiring Ann and Michael to have degrees in surgery.

Underlying the demand for detailed information on surgical technique was perhaps a desperate desire for certainty. Ann and Michael talked with the psychologist about their terror that Tamsin might die this time. If she survived, would she remember the operation and suffer emotionally? Would she blame them later? Their feelings about her appearance resurfaced. How different would she look? They both dreaded not recognizing the daughter they had grown to love, yet secretly hoped her looks would be improved and felt very guilty about this. Ann mentioned for the first time how hard she found it to cope with public reaction when she took Tamsin out. She never knew what to do or say and felt enraged by her own helplessness. How would Tamsin cope with the staring and comments if she herself could not?

There were no easy answers or quick solutions. The first step was providing a secure space for Ann and Michael to voice their uncertainties and terror that, successful surgery or not, the familiar Tamsin might still be lost for ever. They began to discuss the importance of appearance for each of them and what they personally felt about Tamsin's looks.

Michael said he still found it difficult to shake off the self-blame and hurt he carried inside, the feeling that he had caused the facial abnormality. Ann described the shame that welled up when strangers asked about her child and what had happened to her. She said it was so important for them to have produced a normal daughter first, to prove to the world that she could do it. Ann and Michael were to return to this theme many times. For now, they also needed to feel enough control over the surgical proposals to decide whether to accept mid-face surgery for Tamsin. They spoke again with the surgeons and later with the ward sister, this time focusing on what they could expect after the operation rather than on the technique itself.

Tamsin was two-and-a-half years old when she underwent major surgery for the third time. There were postoperative complications but she survived and made a good recovery. Ann and Michael felt enormous relief and delight at Tamsin's new looks, especially since the nasal prong was no longer needed. For the first time in her life, Tamsin resisted infections, gained weight and generally thrived. Ann could now dare to envisage a hospital-free existence for her child and began to look at suitable local playgroups. She felt unsure about what to say to teachers or how to respond when other people reacted to Tamsin's appearance, and requested a meeting with the psychologist at their next outpatient attendance.

This was the first of several sessions in which Ann reflected on the importance that physical attractiveness held for her and the stigma she felt because Tamsin looked so different. As her shame began to grow less and she felt less personally 'attacked' by public gaze, she could start to think about strategies to help herself, and eventually to help Tamsin to deal with unwelcome looks, comments or questions. Tamsin would take her lead from her parents and it was important for them to be as competent and well-rehearsed as possible. Ann considered ways in which she would feel able to react to others (e.g. by deliberately ignoring others by cutting herself off from what was going on around her, by staring back and thus making other people drop their gaze, or by direct comments such as 'my child has Crouzon's syndrome and your staring does not help'). She was taught relaxation techniques that she could use if she ever felt uncomfortably anxious in public. Over several months, Ann reported that she felt like Tamsin's protector, and far less a victim of disfigurement.

By the age of four years, Tamsin was attending a local nursery school with additional help from a teacher for the deaf. She was curious and sociable, and delighted in playing with other children. They were more likely to comment on her hearing aid than on her unusual appearance.

A developmental assessment showed Tamsin was of good intellectual ability; the only delay was to her speech and language as a result of her hearing loss. She may have looked different, but she was an ordinary little girl like everyone else, and Ann and Michael (and Tamsin herself!) made sure no-one forgot that.

There were now long intervals between visits to the outpatient clinic. There would be more surgery in the future, but for now Ann and Michael were concentrating on a busy family life with their daughters. Ann reported that, although young children were initially fearful, they easily accepted her explanations of Tamsin's appearance, once they had been reassured that it was no-one's fault and was not catching. They also recognized that Tamsin could do all that they could do. Tamsin herself had not yet commented on her appearance. Her older sister tended to be overprotective but had bouts of strong jealousy and felt anger towards her parents. Ann and Michael were very aware of how her needs had had to take second place, particularly when Tamsin was in hospital. Michael continued to seem sad and withdrawn at times, but rejected any help for himself. Continued follow-up would be offered throughout Tamsin's childhood and adolescence.

This type of specialist psychological care is generally available within regional centres such as the major craniofacial units. However, there are many families who have babies with diverse congenital problems who do not receive such care. As with all three cases described above, skilled and experienced psychological help allows those with a visible difference and their families to cope more effectively with psychological and social problems.

Chapter 26

Support for professional carers

Nick Ambler

What is support and why is it important?

It is hard to specify the limits of what might be called 'support' in a health care setting. Sometimes, a regular meeting with a supervisor is called a support group. Sometimes it is the discussion that goes on between colleagues over coffee. Nevertheless, most would recognize that having some form of support is a necessity.

In a broad sense, support is a process through which professional carers can develop understanding, skill and resilience in their work. Support helps to maintain people under pressure and to enable them to cope with emotional stress. It can help a team to hold together through a crisis phase. In the absence of support, professional carers are more vulnerable to the psychological hazards of their work.

This chapter is concerned with the nature of emotional strain on professional carers who work in the area of disfigurement. It discusses ways of responding to the challenge this presents. Four steps are suggested for those intending to set up a support process. Finally, there are some comments about crisis situations in which support is most critically needed. This is written mainly for health care professionals. Nevertheless, even if your interest comes from a different perspective you will probably still find aspects of this topic both relevant and useful.

Recognizing emotional strain

Many types of work are physically strenuous. Examples of this range from different forms of labouring through to top-class professional sport. Typically, such work demands a high standard of physical fitness. There is also a need for training, and to understand and follow methods of good practice to avoid causing injury to oneself or to others. It is easily understood that a physically demanding job can be exhausting and that there will be occasions when workers are injured.

Can the same be said of work that is emotionally strenuous? There is evidence of this but it is only quite recently that the idea of emotional strain at work has gained recognition. This has come from studies of so-called 'burnout' in the caring professions.

The notion of a burned out professional is somebody who has reached a stage of emotional exhaustion and has become cynical and cut off from work as a result. It may then be impossible to carry on at work. To do so will probably have adverse effects on both patients and colleagues alike. Maintaining a capacity for dealing with emotional demands is, after all, a basic requirement in the caring professions.

There is presently considerable attention directed towards how to avoid burnout. The concern is the same as with other kinds of occupational hazard. There is a need to prevent the costly loss of trained and valued individuals who provide care. Organizing staff support is considered to be the most appropriate means of prevention.

The term burnout refers only to the extreme end of a range. It would be misleading to concentrate on this alone when considering emotional strain and the kind of support which is needed to offset it. It is more appropriate to look instead at the different signs of emotional strain that arise at an earlier stage, before burnout occurs. Some examples are shown below:

- Tiredness and fatigue;
- Poor sleep;
- Frequent headaches or other pains;
- Heavier drinking or smoking;
- Irritability or quick temper;
- Strains in close relationships;
- Defeatist, fatalistic thinking;
- Distancing from emotional involvement in work;
- Inflexibility: over-reliance on rules, regulations or procedures;
- Difficulty with making decisions;
- Inappropriate humour;
- Overdefensiveness with minor errors or criticisms.

If you recognize most of these in yourself, then you are seriously over-burdened by emotional strain. It is more likely, however, that you will recognize only one or two. This does not mean that you have become burned out. These are simply some of the signs of the emotional demands that arise naturally when working in a caring profession.

Emotional demands related to disfigurement

You will probably have come across colleagues who ask how it is that you can manage to work with patients who have disfigurements. Many people seem intimidated by the thought of what might confront them in this line of work, or even frightened of their own reactions.

Not everyone feels this way. If you have chosen this kind of work, there are likely to have been positive reasons for your decision. For some, it is because they have themselves had personal experience of disfigurement and feel they want to make use of this. Some want to put something back by helping others, having previously been helped themselves. Alternatively, there may have been some appeal in the fact that this is a special and demanding kind of work, which others could not undertake. For some, it is the intensity that makes it particularly attractive. Often, however, the reasons for choosing to work with disfigurement will be more subtle and harder to understand, even in yourself.

In a commentary on the reactions of staff working in a burns unit, Bernstein (1976) described how some doctors experience feelings of shock or morbid curiosity. These were first reactions after joining the burns unit. He also described two popular strategies that helped to overcome these effects. The first was the shifting of attention from the appearance of the burn injuries, to focus instead, on the person and to empathize with their position. The second strategy was simply to build up a daily familiarity with the nature of burns and burned appearances. Regular contact in itself helped to overcome the problem.

Not everyone who works in this area does so through choice. It is mainly those in more senior positions who have chosen to work with people who have disfigurements. If it has become your career, you will already have a daily familiarity with the work and will have developed a means of coping with its particular stresses. For others, however, especially those in training, the prospect of working with disfigured people can be daunting. It can be hard for established and more senior staff to understand this and sympathize with someone newly entering this field of work.

This difference in the level of awareness that professionals have to the impact of disfigurement produces two contrasting problems. The first concerns a heightened sensitivity. New and unaccustomed helpers are more vulnerable because of fears about the personal reactions that this work might provoke. What is needed to compensate for this is a careful and supportive induction course, supervised by experienced staff. This is similar to the care that is needed for patients and relatives at the time of their first encounter following a newly acquired disfigured appearance. Some time is taken beforehand for preparation. The initial encounter may still have unsettling effects but confidence grows as the experience becomes more familiar.

The opposite problem concerns sensitivity that has been lost. If you no longer react to a disfigured appearance when meeting someone for the first time it becomes impossible to understand the significance of their disfigurement. This can be an issue for more experienced helpers. Some develop a more blunted sensitivity to the appearance and predicament of those in their care.

A similar phenomenon has been demonstrated with judgements made by nurses about the level of pain being experienced by patients in a burns unit (Chonière et al., 1990). More experienced nurses underrated the pain when this was compared with patients' own judgements. Less experienced nurses produced closer estimates to those given by their patients. It seemed that length of professional experience actually reduced the nurses' sensitivity. This is a serious concern because nurses rely on this kind of awareness to guide them in carrying out patient care.

The message here is that, whilst the build-up of experience improves a professional carer's self-confidence, it is important to try to preserve some sense of first reaction to meeting each new person who has a disfigurement.

What is meant by support?

There are certain kinds of support, which, although beneficial, are never-theless not the intended subject of this chapter. These include improvements in working conditions, such as better leisure facilities, longer breaks and a safer environment. There are the plans made only for major incidents when, for a brief period, entirely different circumstances prevail. There are staff counselling services that provide help at times of personal emotional crisis. These all amount to a form of support but they are not concerned with the continuous day to day emotional pressures that arise as part of working in a health care environment. An example of support that does tackle this is the type described in an account of a staff group held in a burns and plastics unit (Antebi and Ambler, 1989).

Elsewhere, the different labels given to such arrangements include peer support meetings, clinical supervision, sensitivity groups, professional devel-opment programmes, quality circles, stress management and in-service counselling training for health care staff. Any of these can be used directly to address the emotional demands of the work.

Organizing support

There is wide variation between different professional groups about the priority given to support and the way this is set up. Amongst psychological therapists and social workers, it would be expected that time was routinely set aside for supervision to take account of the emotional strains of their work. For surgeons and physicians, such an arrangement would be extre-mely unusual; whatever arrangements they do make for support tend to be discreet and in their own time.

Even the best arrangements for support can fail. The following steps are suggested as a plan to try to avoid some of the pitfalls.

Step one

Decide on the aims for the support being set up. Examples of these might be:

- To build up a better understanding of psychological reactions;
- To serve as a problem-solving meeting;
- To diffuse tensions within a team;
- To supervise psychological care plans;
- To increase the theoretical knowledge of the participants;
- To resolve the effects of a crisis.

Any or several of these could become the aim of a system of support. Various aims can be tackled using different forms of support (e.g. super-vision meetings to plan patient care plus training events to improve the knowledge base).

Step two: personal preparation

In order to derive any benefit from support, it is important to recognize that it is not a passive process. This means making a time commitment despite other pressures that may exist. One pitfall would be to include people in something which they do not feel they need. This would undermine the process for everyone concerned.

Self-awareness (that is, a willingness to consider your own feelings and reactions) is also fundamental to the process. Initially, this can feel quite awkward if you have always tried to set aside your personal reactions at work.

One particularly important element of self-awareness is to develop an understanding of what you personally derive from your work. You will be able to put up with immense and continuous strains if, in the process, you can still obtain the same satisfaction from it. On the other hand, if you lose the main source of enjoyment in your job, then even the undemanding phases will turn into a strain. It is important to try to take care of the rewarding aspects of work as a professional carer.

Lastly, support requires mutual commitment. It involves sharing with the others who take part, giving as well as receiving help. Those who demand help and support from colleagues, without ever reciprocating, tend eventually to be rejected. Even those who attend, but who say little and therefore do not become involved, will also become left out of the support process.

Step three: find the supporters

Support can be developed in many forms and can involve different people. They might be people with whom you have no other working contact. It might be the whole team in which you work. One pitfall is if this combines both junior and senior members of a managerial hierarchy. It is difficult for either to reveal their uncertainties and insecurities about their work. This will put a block on the use of a meeting for personal emotional support. Finding an outside facilitator, who is not involved in any other way with a team may get around this, adding both a sense of security and respect for the support process. Alternatively, it is possible to tease out different aspects of support. A team can arrange some parts to be undertaken together, while personal emotional support could be set up elsewhere.

Step four: maintain the commitment

Numerous staff support meetings are set up at a time of crisis and then fizzle out after the situation has calmed down. Stress management events are an example. One or two sessions might be hurriedly organized in the face of demands for better support. One-off arrangements are quickly forgotten afterwards; on their own, they are insufficient to deal with a more general need for support.

Another pitfall concerns attendance. Those people involved in a support process need to take part consistently. Occasional and unreliable contributions do not work.

Another way in which support can break down is because of the low priority it takes when there is greater pressure at work. You may feel inclined to make more work time available by pulling out of a support arrangement. Ironically, this will take away the very means through which you might cope more effectively during periods of increased stress.

Responding to crises

Occasionally, a turn of events can put a team of health care staff into turmoil. The unexpected death of a patient, a serious error by a member of the team, an assault on a member of staff, a serious complaint by a patient, a grievance or dispute amongst colleagues, or even the departure of the team leader or another valued member of staff.

Any event that provokes unusual pressures will test the resources and support that exist within a team. If these are already stretched to the limits, then such a situation can trigger serious after-effects. Examples of these effects are high levels of sickness and absenteeism, deteriorating team performance and staff deciding to leave.

On the other hand, several characteristics of a good system of support will enable a team to work through such periods of increased pressure. Three examples are as follows:

First, supervision can help with crisis prevention. It will help you to judge how much you can take on. For example, if a patient has become seriously emotionally disturbed, it is not always clear how and when an outside specialist should be called in. Regular supervision should clarify the level of distress that the team can reasonably tackle with a patient, as well as the stage when referral to a specialist is required. This is sometimes described as the issue of boundaries. An understanding of boundaries helps individuals to avoid getting out of depth with their work. It also prevents a whole team from allowing a situation to deteriorate too far before requesting outside help. An awareness of limits will also improve liaison with the outside specialists. If the referrals they receive are more appropriate and better timed they are less likely to feel 'dumped-on', as would be the case when a problem has reached a crisis level. Supervision and clear reasoning about boundaries therefore go some way towards averting such crises.

Secondly, an effective system of support encourages you to be aware of the signs of emotional strain in yourself and in those working alongside you. You learn to pace yourself against the demands made on you. When the effects of personal strain are starting to emerge, there is then the back-up of knowing that this is more likely to draw helpful reactions from colleagues. In a less supportive atmosphere at a time when you may be experiencing particular strain, there is no such help to fall back on when required.

Thirdly, a well-organized system of support has flexibility. During crisis phases, it is possible to make special arrangements to respond to the extra pressure. For example, the unexpected death of a patient might lead a team to arrange a meeting quickly in order to talk through what has occurred. Such meetings are often used to reorganize and wind down in reaction to a crisis. However, in the absence of a familiar support process, it is less clear who should organize such a meeting. Also, having previously had little experience of this, the participants will be unsure about what happens and less able to make good use of it. There are no such problems for those who regularly meet to discuss the psychological pressures provoked by their work.

A crisis faced by a health care team is often a catalyst for organizing better support in future. This happens because the event serves to highlight deficiencies that previously existed. Some might regard this as an example of learning the hard way. Conversely, however, a crisis can underline just how well a system of support has been working. If, at the end, there is a shared sense of having coped effectively, then this will be a boost to staff morale. Reacting well to crises, therefore, has the longer-term benefit of strengthening a professional team.

Making the case for staff support

It has been assumed throughout this chapter that, whatever the system of staff support you are using or trying to set up, it will be properly recognized as part of your work. This is described as 'formal support'. In practice, examples of formal support in medical and surgical settings are rare. What exists in its place is usually 'informal', that is, an ad hoc arrangement between individuals carried out in their own time.

Why should this be so?

Formal support promises tangible benefits, such as the improved morale, performance and retention of staff. This enhances the quality of patient care. A problem is that it is often difficult to persuade managers and senior medical staff about the need for formal support. After all, it does appear to reduce the time staff have available for their patients. You will need to present a strong case with evidence. It is usually necessary to carry out a survey of staff stress to demonstrate the problem objectively. If so, there are a variety of standardized questionnaires that have been designed for this purpose. The most widely recognized is the Maslach scale (Maslach and Jackson, 1981).

Managers regard staff morale as a responsibility for which they are accountable. If they are confronted with survey results that describe failings in this area, they will probably feel criticized and defensive. It is more effective to involve a senior figure at the beginning of the process of evaluating the need for staff support.

Another possible barrier is that managers and senior medical staff will almost certainly work under high stress themselves. This may well be in circumstances where support is even less accessible and where this would be seen as a sign of weakness or dependency. If the manager is stressed and unsupported, then he or she may well give a negative reaction to proposals about formal support for other staff.

There are other sources of information that can help you to prepare a case. In the UK, the National Association for Staff Support provides both information and practical advice. They also run a helpline for nurses (see the end of this chapter for addresses). The King's Fund has produced guidelines for the clinical supervision of nurses (Kohner, 1994). In 1992, the British Medical Association published a report on stress amongst doctors, which is helpful in formulating a proposal.

Finally, there is now health and safety legislation in the UK directed at employers to ensure that their staff are not exposed to excessive psychological stress without reasonable arrangements being made to offset the effects (Cox and Cox, 1993). It is hoped that this legislation will drive forward the development of formal support, with improved arrangements being implemented widely across different health care settings.

References

Antebi, D. and Ambler, N. (1989). A staff group in a burns unit: managing patients' psychological needs. *Psychiatr. Bull.,* **13**, 65–66.

Bernstein, N. R. (1976). *The Emotional Care of the Facially Burned and Disfigured.* Boston: Little Brown.

British Medical Association. (1992). *Stress and the Medical Profession.* London: BMA.

Chonière M., Melzack R., Girard N., Rondeau J. and Paquin M–J. (1990). Comparisons between patients' and nurses' assessment of pain and medication efficacy in severe burn injuries. *Pain,* **40**, 143–152.

Cox, T. and Cox, S. (1993). Occupational health: control and monitoring of psychosocial and organisational hazards at work. *J. R. Soc. Health,* **113**, 201–205.

Kohner, N. (1994). *Clinical Supervision in Practice.* London: King's Fund. (126 Albert Street, London NW1 7NF, UK.)

Maslach, C. and Jackson, S. E. (1981). The measurement of experienced burn-out. *J. Occup. Behav.,* **2**, 91–113.

Information sources

National Association for Staff Support, 9 Caradon Close, Woking, Surrey, UK.
'Nurseline': a helpline for nurses and midwifes. Tel: 0181 681 4030.

Chapter 27

The role of support groups

James Partridge and Poppy Nash

Introduction

Having considered the nature and range of the professional help available to the visibly different patient, this chapter will offer a glimpse at the variety of ways in which patients can help themselves and each other in coming to terms with their circumstances by means of self-support or self-help organizations. For the purposes of this chapter, they will be called self-help organizations or groups, since this describes exactly what they aim to be; that is, self-helping rather than reliant on professional and external support. In a few cases, the groups may be set up and led by a professional.

The term 'organization' will be used here to describe a formally constituted body with employees. In contrast, the term 'group' will imply a voluntary association of interested people. 'Self-help bodies' will refer to both types.

Self-help organizations/groups can be defined as entities that are run by and for the benefit of those with a visible difference (often a facial disfigurement) or their parents, or by people who are going through or have been through the same or a similar experience.

The role of self-help bodies differs according to how the organizers see the most appropriate means of reaching their common purposes. Broadly, they all aim to enhance the quality of life of their members, whether they are drawn from a wide geographical area (e.g. the whole country) or a much more defined group (such as the local burns unit).

In pursuing this aim, self-help groups/organizations become involved in a whole range of activities including:

- Socializing within the group and with professionals;
- Specific activities (such as going to the swimming baths);
- Hospital visiting of patients;
- Regular closed group meetings;
- Information-giving;
- Networking of others suffering the same difficulty;
- Emotional support by phone, letter or in person;
- Therapeutic activities of various kinds;
- Advocacy;

- Lobbying and campaigning;
- Other educational work;
- Fund raising for research or other objectives.

Some organizations attempt to offer a large number of these, others concentrate entirely on one only. Most groups have a local focus and quite naturally are not resourced to provide a long list of activities. A full list of UK self-help organizations is provided at the end of this chapter.

The diversity of memberships and structures

Although the organizations/groups are primarily run to offer support to those with a visible difference, their members may include professionals working in the field of disfigurement and the families of children with disfigurements. This diversity of membership can both help and hinder the establishment of an effective supportive group. In some instances, a local group will be run by ex-patients, a professional committed to self-help initiatives, or a combination of the two depending upon where the group meetings are held.

Issues that frequently involve much discussion amongst group members concern where and when the meetings should take place; the options include day, evening or weekend meetings. Whilst those who are not employed may favour daytime meetings, this is often not feasible for members who are employed. The best venue can also generate discussion, since some members may wish to meet outside the hospital environment, whilst others may prefer to meet within it. Geographical distance can also play a major role in deciding how the group is run.

A small number of national self-help organizations has been established to provide psychological/social support to facially disfigured people and their families. These groups produce regular newsletters or bulletins to keep their members abreast of the organizations' activities and other initiatives. Some have raised significant funds for their endeavours.

The *Disfigurement Guidance Centre* (DGC) in Cupar, Fife, was the first such organization set up in the UK. Founded by Doreen Trust, who has written several books on her experience of living with a port-wine stain, the DGC has run courses and offered help to many parents and other individuals (especially those with birthmarks) since its launch in the mid-1960s. It has also campaigned actively for more laser therapy units to be set up in the NHS and has raised over £1 million for lasers to be bought and installed in NHS hospitals (through the LaserFair campaign).

Let's Face It (LFI) is another national support network for the facially disfigured population. Set up by Mrs Christine Piff after her experience of facial cancer, LFI was founded in 1983 and is now a registered charity. It offers support and companionship for people with a facial disfigurement, especially after hospital discharge following cancer treatment. Local branches of this organization have been set up around the country with a variety of arrangements about where and when the regular meetings are held. An annual garden party is held at which the friendships are established and renewed.

Changing Faces is a relatively new charity which seeks to help facially disfigured people to live with greater confidence, and to reduce the general public's ignorance and fear of disfigurement. It was founded by James Partridge after the reception given to his book of the same name. Over the past three years, *Changing Faces* has pioneered a new programme of rehabilitation for facially disfigured people, which has focused upon enhancing social skills, such as how to cope with other people's reactions to disfigurement. In mastering these essential skills, members feel a growing sense of self-confidence and ability to handle challenging situations. The charity has gained some significant financial backing and employs professional staff who are specialists in this field; it is now supported by a core grant from the Department of Health.

Two other condition-specific organizations merit brief mention as examples of the diversity of national self-help activity. The *National Eczema Society* is a very large provider of information and organizer of courses about this very common skin condition. The *Cleft Lip and Palate Association* (CLAPA) has grown from a very small parent support group to a thriving organization with over 30 local branches and plans to become even more solidly constructed in the future.

Alongside the national organizations exist a variety of self-help groups, which function independently of the national networks. Examples of these include the *Face to Face* self-help group for the facially disfigured, which meets at the Walton Hospital in Liverpool, and the *Burns Support Group*, which is based in Sheffield.

Since self-help bodies serve such a diverse range of needs of their individual members, there are bound to be a variety of models of practice. Local groups attached to a particular hospital unit have many advantages over the bigger organizations but there are some drawbacks too. The rest of this chapter seeks to identify those pros and cons.

The benefits of self-help organizations

Whilst there are numerous and unquestionable benefits of belonging to a self-help group/organization, the most notable are highlighted below.

- The support body can offer the patient/ex-patient a unique forum for meeting other people who are experiencing similar difficulties and hospital treatment. Supportive and nurturing friendships can be established, which may be sustained long after the person has been officially discharged from hospital.
- Where the self-help body is a nurturing one, the empathy and understanding it provides to its members can encourage the development of adaptive coping skills and appropriate social skills. For example, a person's damaged self-esteem and self-confidence can be gradually restored, thus equipping him or her with the essential psychological 'survival kit' to lead an independent and fulfilling life.
- If the group/organization is well established, it may be in a position to give individual support throughout the period of hospital treatment and beyond. For instance, a person may benefit from group membership at

the preoperative and postoperative stages and after hospital discharge. Depending upon its primary function, it may be able to offer different forms of support at different junctures of the person's treatment, starting from the time of the initial diagnosis or onset (where applicable). When the disfigurement is present at birth, the group can play a crucial role in supporting the patient's parents. In similar vein, where the disfigurement is acquired in later life, the group can offer a supportive hand to the patient's partner. Thus, self-help organizations extend a welcome to close members of the patient's family.

- Some self-help bodies may also be in a position to offer inpatient support and to counsel in preparing for discharge into the 'outside' world. The transition from hospital to home may seem especially threatening and daunting to those with a facial disfigurement, and, therefore, support in this area can be invaluable to long-term and satisfactory adjustment.
- The individual members of a self-help group/organization can collectively create an environment in which it is 'safe' to explore thoughts and feelings about experiences of everyday life. In encouraging the expression of anxieties in a nonjudgemental and accepting arena, the individual can be helped to face his or her particular difficulties without fear of rejection or derision, thereby diminishing common tendencies to deny and/or avoid areas of awkwardness and embarrassment. In that such activities can directly address the problems encountered by the members of the organization, the group can be seen as playing a broadly therapeutic and counselling role. The role of the 'leader' of the group is a crucial one and some have benefited significantly from attending counselling/group-leading courses.
- A self-help body may have an explicitly social role. In this instance, the group network may have a calendar of social events to which members and their partners (or parents in the case of children) are invited. In other instances, an organization may foster both therapeutic and social roles, depending upon the needs of the individual members at any given time.
- Some self-help groups/organizations are committed to pursuing an educational role by sharing knowledge, giving information and acting as a resource for those wishing to discover more about facial disfigurement. Amongst their activities are the production of literature for local and/or national distribution, producing a newsletter or bulletin on a regular basis, and engaging in media publicity, such as newspaper and television coverage.
- Self-help bodies may additionally be involved in fund raising for the purpose of research or purchasing equipment to enable new treatment methods, such as laser surgery, to be made available.

Taken together, these points put forward a strong case for recommending membership of a self-help organization to any patient/ex-patient. However, the choice regarding membership must be based on a very clear assessment of what the group can offer to each prospective member. For example, it is quite inappropriate for somebody seeking emotional support to get in touch with an organization that is primarily involved in research funding. Equally, as another example, somebody who is seeking information about local services and living in the north, cannot be expected to be enthusiastic about joining a group that operates at the other end of the country. Indeed, to be of any value, membership of a group/organization must be both practicable and viable, since membership usually generates a strong commitment from its members.

There is a growing need for a nationally co-ordinated information service to provide details on the state of the art regarding the sources of support available to disfigured people. *Changing Faces* is developing a national information centre, which may serve as a valuable central resource point.

The potential problems of self-help groups/organizations

The potential problems to be outlined in this section are considered from the perspective of the (ex-)patient and his or her family. Whilst the merits of self-help groups are indisputable as well as diverse, in reality, the ideal is not always realized for a variety of reasons. Therefore, in order to paint a balanced picture, the potential drawbacks of these groups need to be considered alongside their obvious benefits:

- In some situations, professionals may feel uncomfortable and reluctant to become involved with a self-help organization (even if the meetings are hospital-based). The main objections may include the fear of becoming too personally involved with patients, or the fear that patients may become too dependent upon them or the hospital staff in general, once treatment has been completed. Another common perception held by professionals is that people who meet together because they share similar symptoms or disease, reinforce a role of passivity by comparing experiences and problems. This contrasts with the notion of the active patient who strives to face the challenge of disfigurement without being conceivably 'fuelled' by others' anxieties.
- Self-help organizations may be considered to provide the therapeutic 'treatment' that the professionals cannot or do not provide due to lack of resources and time pressures. In this way, professionals may be perceived as 'off-loading' their responsibilities on to members of the group. An example of this might be the member who offers to visit an inpatient at the preoperative stage to try to allay some of that person's anxieties about the forthcoming surgery.
- Self-help organizations are often run on the goodwill and enthusiasm of its members. Whilst this is laudable, awkward situations can arise when a member wishes to visit new patients on the hospital ward prior to surgery or to meet new members, when they are not really the best people to do so (for whatever reason). Thus, the professionals may feel that a system of careful vetting is required, which by its very nature carries implications of suitability and value judgement. This situation may be compounded by the fact that the potential visitor considers himself or herself to be uniquely suited to the task, since he or she has experienced the same or similar surgery. It is exactly because each person's circumstances are different, that the anticipation of the same treatment outcome can hamper rather than help such a relationship.

- Where the primary activity of a self-help group is social in nature, there can be a dilemma for professionals involved in the group. That is, the problem of accountability can arise when the group welcomes professional involvement, but does not warrant their professional time in terms of requiring therapeutic help.
- Whilst it is invaluable in some cases for the family and friends of patients/ ex-patients to participate in group activities (whether social or therapeutic in nature), their involvement can exert an adverse influence upon the dynamics and focus of the group. For example, attention may be turned to the personal problems of families and friends rather than upon the group members themselves. Although caring for the carers is a very important part of the whole process of adjustment, on some occasions it may be necessary to review for whom the self-help organization exists.
- There may be a tendency for the self-help group to attract certain personality types amongst the facially disfigured population. This can cause vulnerable members to feel threatened or overwhelmed by more outgoing and gregarious members. In such instances, sensitivity is clearly required, since the group may be serving individuals' needs in different ways.
- It is important to ask how professional involvement in a self-help group/ organization (if applicable) may affect the patient–professional relationship, especially when the patient is still receiving hospital treatment supervised by the professional concerned.
- When a person is receiving a lengthy programme of hospital-based treatment, an attachment to the hospital may develop, which is founded on the patient's deep sense of gratitude to the hospital, or on a feeling of resentment that the desired results have not been realized. If the self-help group meets within the hospital, it can encourage a sense of dependency on the establishment, which may be disadvantageous to those concerned. Indeed, sometimes the hospital is perceived as a 'family' to which the patient feels he or she belongs. Whilst this view may reflect the nurturing offered by the hospital staff, it is not a healthy perception to harbour for life.
- A further question to address regarding self-help organizations, is the extent to which they convey messages of 'normality' and 'pathology' to their members. In the former case, the potential psychosocial difficulties associated with facial disfigurement may be minimized, whereas in the latter case, the import of such difficulties may be exaggerated. Thus, an organization must be sensitive to both dimensions and attempt to convey a balanced and realistic ideology.
- Continuing the theme of sensitivity, the self-help group may appear very daunting to those who are feeling vulnerable, and/or those who are not yet ready to join in the activities. Such people may easily take a 'back seat' and become relatively neglected, when it is they who may be especially in need of the benefits of group membership.
- The actual size of self-help groups may reflect the extent to which it has become a 'closed shop'. There is a clear distinction between the group that genuinely welcomes new members, and thereby encourages its membership to grow, and the group that enjoys a more clique-like existence, characterized by members who know each other well, and a reluctance to expand. This reluctance may suggest that potential expansion is threatening to the group who have invested trust in each other.

- A potential drawback concerning self-help groups may be a lack of consensus amongst members about the primary objective of the group. For instance, whilst some may see it as a vehicle for challenging policy regarding treatment and related issues, others may believe that social support should be the group's main priority. With sensitive handling, these differences of opinion can be resolved, but in some cases they may herald fundamental obstacles to the group's growth and development. In view of this, honest and open discussion amongst members about the function of the group can help to forestall such problems.

The link that is made between hospital staff (and perhaps GPs) and local self-help groups is vital, since these professionals are in a position to recommend local groups, or indeed national organizations, to their patients. Far too infrequently are patients given information about supportive organizations that are outside the arena of statutory health services. There seems to be disquiet amongst some professionals, especially plastic surgeons, about the work of some self-help groups or organizations. This is mainly due to the perceived interference by organizers of these groups in the treatment options and decision making upon which the surgeon has embarked. With greater communication and liaison between professionals and the self-help organizations, such perceptions can be checked.

Summary

Self-help groups/organizations not only play an enormously valuable role for their individual members, but they can also be regarded as a force for change. That is, they can function as a pressure group that will increase the accountability, quality of care and resources provided to enable and empower patients to live with their visible difference in an effective and positive way.

In today's world, where the public services are under increasing pressure, self-help organizations provide a vital link between the formal hospital services and the more spread-eagled and often unco-ordinated social services. It may well be the case that this type of organization often provides a service that would not otherwise be available.

Disfigurement support organizations

ACNE SUPPORT GROUP
PO Box 230, Hayes, Middlesex UB4 0UT
Tel: 0181 561 686
Provides up-to-date information about acne and rosacea, and has a newsletter
Founded by Dr Tony Chu, a dermatologist, in 1993

BACUP
3 Bath Place, Rivington Street, London EC2A 3JR
Tel: Info: 0800 181199 or 0171 613 2121; Counselling: 0171 696 9000

Provides professional information by phone and leaflet on many aspects of cancer, and has a counselling service for those who can reach its base
Founded in the early 1980s by Dr Vicki Clement-Jones, a GP who later died of cancer

CANCERLINK
11–21 Northdown Street, London N1 9BN
Tel: 0171 833 2451
Provides information and networking for groups and individuals affected by cancer; runs courses and workshops on all aspects of cancer care and self-help

CHANGING FACES
1 and 2 Junction Mews, Paddington, London W2 1PN
Tel: 0171 706 4232
Provides information and advice, counselling and social skills workshops in London and around Britain for anyone affected by facial disfigurement whatever the cause
Founded by James Partridge, a burns survivor, in 1992

CLEFT LIP AND PALATE ASSOCIATION (CLAPA)
Head Office, 134 Buckingham Palace Road, London SW1 9SA
Tel: 0171 824 8110
Has a national network of local parent support groups and provides supportive literature and aids to help with feeding etc.
Founded by staff at Great Ormond Street Hospital

CRANIOFACIAL SUPPORT GROUP
44 Helmsdale Road, Leamington Spa, Warks CV32 7DW
Tel: 01926 334629
Newly established in 1994 to provide a network of families with craniofacial conditions such as Apert's and Crouzon's syndromes

CYSTIC HYGROMA SUPPORT GROUP
Mrs Pearl Fowler, Villa Fontana, Church Road, Crawley, West Sussex
Tel: 01293 885901
Provides information about the condition and contact with other families; organizes an all-day meeting once a year

DISFIGUREMENT GUIDANCE CENTRE
PO Box 7, Cupar, Fife KY15 4PF
Tel: 01337 870281
Provides information and advice, especially concerning birthmarks, and raises money for laser therapy via the charity, Laser Fair
Founded in the 1960s by Doreen Trust who has a portwine stain

DISFIGUREMENT INTEREST GROUP
Dr Nichola Rumsey, Department of Psychology, University of the West of England, St Mathias, Fishponds, Bristol, Avon BS16 2JP
Tel: 0117 9655384
A multidisciplinary group of professionals working and researching in the area of visible difference

DISFIGUREMENT SUPPORT UNIT (OUTLOOK)
Frenchay Hospital, Bristol, Avon BS16 1LE

DYSTROPHIC EPIDERMOLYSIS BULLOSA RESEARCH ASSOCIATION (DEBRA)
Debra House, 13 Wellington Business Park, Dukes Ride, Crowthorne, Berkshire RG45 6LS
Tel: 01344 771961
Provides information and newsletters, has full-time support nurses and raises funds for medical research

LET'S FACE IT
14 Fallowfield, Yateley, Surrey GU17 7LU
Tel: 01252 879630
Provides a support network around the UK and in other countries for those with facial disfigurements, especially after cancer treatment; has a summer garden party
Founded by Christine Piff in 1983 after her experience of facial cancer

LUPUS UK
1 Eastern Road, Romford, Essex RM1 3NH
Tel: 01708 731251
Provides support and contact through local groups, advice and information as well as organizing educational meetings

NAEVUS SUPPORT GROUP
58 Necton Road, Wheathampstead, St Albans, Herts
Tel: 01582 832853
Provides information about all forms of birthmark and a support network of parents meets twice a year
Founded and run by Renate and John O'Neill

NATIONAL ECZEMA SOCIETY
163 Eversholt Street, London NW1 1BU
Tel: 0171 388 4097
Provides information and advice on many aspects of eczema for parents and professionals; campaigns for more resources within the NHS and has educational aims

NEUROFIBROMATOSIS ASSOCIATION (LINK)
82 London Road, Kingston upon Thames, Surrey KT2 6PX
Tel: 0181 547 1636
Information, contact with other parents, support and advice; newsletter and meetings

THE PSORIASIS ASSOCIATION
7 Milton Street, Northampton NN2 7JG
Tel: 01604 711129
Provides a range of information leaflets, newsletters, help and advice and has regional groups around the country

STURGE–WEBER FOUNDATION (UK)
Burleigh, 348 Pinhoe Road, Exeter EX4 8AF

Tel: 01392 464675
Provides support, information and advice to families affected by the condition and has an annual family conference

TREACHER–COLLINS FAMILY SUPPORT GROUP
c/o Sue Moore, 114 Vincent Road, Thorpe Hamlet, Norwich, Norfolk NR1 4HH
Tel: 01603 433736
Provides support, friendship, information and advice on this condition as well as Nager syndrome, and First and Second Arch syndromes

THE VITILIGO SOCIETY
PO Box 919, London SE21 8AW
Tel: 0181 776 7022
Provides support and advice, a regular newsletter and holds meetings to which professionals are invited; also sponsors medical research

OTHER GROUPS
The Guinea Pig Club, c/o Queen Victoria Hospital, East Grinstead, West Sussex RH19 3DZ
National Association of Laryngectomy Clubs, Ground Floor, 6, Rickett Street, London SW6 1RU
British Red Cross – Cosmetic Camouflage Service, 9 Grosvenor Crescent, London SW1X 7EJ

Chapter 28

Conclusion: the way forward

Richard Lansdown, Nichola Rumsey, Nicholas Ambler, David Harris, Poppy Nash, Section Editors and other members of the Disfigurement Interest Group

Introduction

This chapter pulls together themes that have emerged from this book and spells out the implications for policy and practice. In times of financial stringency and political controversy there is a temptation to focus on costs and competing markets but, apart from a passing reference towards the end, this has been resisted. We attempt rather to develop a consistent professional model of understanding and care, keeping the needs of visibly different patients and quality of care in mind as a priority.

One theme that has been discussed and illustrated in Section Two is that current care provision has not, by and large, taken account of what is known from theory and research. The reasons for the lack of dissemination of those findings that have been available in the literature for some years now will become clear in the rest of this chapter. Two points are of the utmost importance.

One is the faulty perception by many professionals of psychosocial needs. Some seem to imagine that all people with disfigurements are 'pathological'. Others are misled by people who put on a brave metaphorical face to hide the pain caused by their real appearance. These people seem to be coping, they are perhaps a little quiet and passive, but they are not aggressive and do not abuse alcohol or drugs. One may wonder just why it is that they are so normal (to paraphrase the title of a research article on clefts) and one may miss the distress that is so carefully hidden. Equally misperceived is the notion that once surgery is completed there is no longer a need for help.

The second point is central to all three sections of this book, and fundamental to our understanding of assessment and treatment. More than most, if not all, other groups who seek health care, the disfigured are a mixed bunch: in their physical characteristics; in their reasons for coming into the health care system; in their medical and surgical needs; and in their psychosocial profiles. Compared with others, it is much harder to predict what the timing and form of their social tensions may be. What is more, there are still grey areas to be explored in the field of the optimal timing of surgery.

An example of the results of this emphasis on the idiosyncratic, as discussed in Section Two, is the way that self-help groups seem to be less successful for those with visible disfigurements than they are for others.

Instead of providing mutual support and a forum for constructive thinking, they can end in unhelpful discontent.

This leads to tension in thinking and planning. On the one hand we are arguing for a consistent model of understanding and care, but on the other we say that we must take account of individual variation. Perhaps this conflict lies behind the failure so far to develop an adequate model.

A comprehensive assessment

One uncontroversial outcome of this variation is the acknowledgement of the necessity for comprehensive assessment which, in turn, means the setting up of a multidisciplinary team.

From one point of view, the setting up of such a team is easy. First, the functions that are going to be required must be decided. In the case of the facially disfigured, they can be grouped into three components:

- The structural remediation component comprises all those who intervene at a physical level by surgery or laser treatment.
- The functional component includes speech and language therapists, occupational therapists, physiotherapists and audiologists.
- The psychosocial component includes psychologists, psychiatrists, social workers and counsellors. The specialist nurse can be included here although he or she could also be included above.

That was the easy part. It is harder to find people to fill these roles. Disfigurement is not one of the glamorous specialties. It does not easily attract research funding. It is, however, immensely rewarding for the few who undertake it.

Even harder is the organization of a team. Generally speaking, the more similar the work done the greater the danger of rivalry between individuals, professions and groups. As two psychologists, the Managing Editors can attest to this occurring when there is overlap between the roles of psychologists and psychiatrists, psychologists and counsellors, or even different types of psychologist. A key figure, then, is the team co-ordinator, someone who will command respect from everyone else while threatening no-one. Personality, commitment and available time are all essential characteristics of this function.

Once the team has been assembled and organized, there needs to be considerable thought given to the ways in which the nature of the needs of the disfigured determine the day to day set-up of an assessment session. Above all, there should be active and equal participation, with, at times, the patient driving the interchange. Medical settings, even today, can be conducive to the imposition of a submissive role on patients; if this does occur, it is so much harder to convey what one thinks and feels rather than what one imagines the doctor wants to hear. Because so many of the needs of the visibly disfigured are not evident to formal tests or observation – there is no radiograph for anguish – it is easy to miss much that should be explored.

One way to facilitate easy communication is to arrange that patients are seen by only one professional at a time. As was discussed in Section Three, a system that allows someone to respond in a small-scale setting is far more likely to facilitate openness than the conventional 'fish bowl' (see Chapter 22). It is more expensive in terms of time but, as we have said, the model we are putting forward is driven by patient needs, not those of the accountant.

Continuity of care

Continuity of care invariably needs to extend beyond the health care setting. This partly involves simple liaison between a hospital and the primary care team in the community, simply so that each knows what the other is doing, has done and plans to do in the future, and, partly, there is an advocacy role to play: teachers and local social workers may need help to understand the sequelae of disfigurement.

It is easier to point to the need for continuity than it is to say how it should be organized, for local conditions will determine local provision. As with the multidisciplinary team in a hospital, appropriate support should be initiated and if possible co-ordinated by one professional who is able to act in a link/liaison capacity. Where that person is based is less important than the capacity to communicate easily across the board.

Community support

Support may need to take a variety of forms. The charity *Changing Faces* has established a pilot Disfigurement Support Unit (DSU), which, although hospital-based, aims to act as a regional centre in the south-west of England, offering information to those with visible differences and their families and friends. Two psychologists are also available to offer psychosocial support and intervention. Referrals are accepted from a variety of sources, including GPs and social workers. The concept of an 'outreach worker' has also been established; this is someone to provide a link between the hospital-based team, the staff of the DSU and the patient in the community. With the patient's permission, the outreach worker can act as an educator, offering information and addressing the concerns of colleagues in the workplace, peers and teachers at school, and family members.

Despite the reservations expressed above about self-help groups, they might also be useful sources of support. Currently however, such groups are fragmented (see Chapter 27). They cannot, therefore, wield much influence and are unable to publicize themselves effectively. The integration of self-help groups into one cohesive organization would seem to promise several benefits. Such an umbrella organization would be able to exert stronger consumer pressure on health care providers to develop a more appropriate and comprehensive service and on those responsible for the allocation of resources to fund services adequately. This could also act as a pressure group to stimulate and fund research.

Professional groups

Some multidisciplinary professional groups exist (for example the Craniofacial Society of Great Britain), but at the moment they tend to focus on a small part of the whole field. The establishment of a national professional body with multidisciplinary membership of those working in the broad field of disfigurement has the potential to provide much needed impetus in a number of key areas. Such an organization would do much to increase the awareness both of members and of the general public about issues relating to the 'syndrome' of visible difference. It would facilitate the pooling of relevant knowledge and would serve an educative function for professionals from different disciplines. In learning about the effectiveness of the interventions that different disciplines can contribute, the efficacy of a multidisciplinary team approach would become apparent. This model could then be promoted in preference to a situation in which a collection of professionals work in isolation and ignorance of each other's capabilities.

A national organization would act as a stimulus to further research, and would promote the desirability of peer review and critical evaluation of the outcome of treatment and interventions. An additional spin-off might be to encourage other professionals to seek to specialize in an area that is currently understaffed by those with relevant interest and expertise.

Walls around the disfigured

It is possible to conceptualize the current situation as one in which a series of walls have been constructed around the person who is considered to be visibly different; walls that form a barrier to and from the majority of the population.

The walls have been created in several ways. Some have been built by the prevailing culture. In a variety of pervasive ways (see Chapters 12 and 15), our society promotes the desirability of physical 'wholeness'. Myths and stereotypes associate physical attractiveness with better prospects for happy and successful lives. They lead to stigmas associated with looking different, and serve to reinforce pre-existing tendencies to form impressions of others based on the way they look.

Some walls result from the way in which care is offered and provided. They reflect the prevailing ethos of the medical model, the aim of care being to restore function, to 'normalize' a person's physical appearance, with too little focus on individual need and psychosocial support.

Walls have been created through the lack of priority attached to visible difference in the allocation of resources, a pattern that seems set to harden. As we have mentioned already, work in this field lacks the drama and obvious appeal of many specialties and the extent and depth of need has not hitherto been appreciated by those responsible for allocating funds.

Other barriers have been constructed by those with visible differences themselves. These result from assumptions (which may be based on negative past experiences) that other people reject them, that they are worthless because they do not look 'right', and that they do not have other means at their disposal to gain control of social situations.

Dismantling the walls

How then might the walls be dismantled? There are both short and longer-term aims to consider. Education clearly has a role to play – in a variety of forms – to increase levels of awareness of the causes and varieties of disfigurement and of how it feels to look different from other people. Education and appropriate training are also required for both purchasers and providers involved in the assessment and treatment of those with a visible difference. A more-broadly based dissemination of information relating to the problem-support facilities that are available can only bring benefits, to the people with disfigurement, their families and friends, and professionals in the field.

These then are the long-term aims, but what of the short term? What can be done in the context of current care provision and acute shortage of funding in many areas of health care? Immediate steps could be taken to rectify the current fragmentation and lack of co-ordination of services. With greater awareness of the needs of patients, it should, in most instances, be possible to harness existing resources into a more coherent framework. As part of this process, current providers of care may be able to evaluate the service they offer by asking themselves some key questions:

- How do we communicate with the patients who come to see us? Is it a one way process? Are the patients and/or the family encouraged to voice their concerns, address a broad spectrum of issues, discuss options in care, or question the extent of the service provision available?
- How effective is the communication with other professionals concerning the care and progress of the patient?
- Is an appropriate and comprehensive assessment carried out?
- How often does an assessment incorporate the psychosocial as well as the 'structural' and 'functional' elements?
- On what basis has the assessment and treatment offered to the patient been developed? Is it up to date? Has it been informed by current research and knowledge in the area?
- Does the service have someone acting in a co-ordinating capacity? Is this person in a position to provide the link with community services, or the school/workplace if necessary? Does this person act as a contact point for the patient and the family?
- Is there a staff support system?
- Is there any audit or critical evaluation of the outcome of care? Does this take account of the view of the patient?

Conclusion

Above all, there is a need to increase professional health workers' awareness of needs in this area and of ways of meeting them. If such an understanding were achieved, there might be a hope of redressing the lack of balance between need and provision. The number of people specializing in this field is tiny – yet between 2% and 3% of the population is affected. After all, if professionals do not understand the nature of visible differences, what hope is there that understanding can be expected among the general public?

In writing this book we hope that we have been able to contribute to an increased awareness of the needs of the visibly different among both professionals and interested members of the general public. This has to be the way forward.

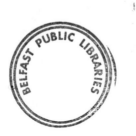

Index